Uveitis in the Clinic - Current Approaches and Future Directions in Diagnosis, Treatment, and Patient Care

Edited by Joobin Khadamy

Published in London, United Kingdom

Uveitis in the Clinic - Current Approaches and Future Directions in Diagnosis, Treatment, and Patient Care
http://dx.doi.org/10.5772/intechopen.1006762
Edited by Joobin Khadamy

Contributors
Flavio Cassano, Gianluca Besozzi, Joobin Khadamy, Maria Carmela Costa, Michele Santoro, Milena L'Abbate, Mustafa Kayabaşı, Noor Ul Ain, Roha Ahmad Choudhary, Seema Rani, Seher Köksaldı, Tayyaba Gul Malik

First published in London, United Kingdom, 2025 by IntechOpen
IntechOpen is the global imprint of INTECHOPEN LIMITED, registered in England and Wales, registration number: 11086078, 167-169 Great Portland Street, London, W1W 5PF, United Kingdom

For EU product safety concerns: IN TECH d.o.o., Prolaz Marije Krucifikse Kozulić 3, 51000 Rijeka, Croatia, info@intechopen.com or visit our website at intechopen.com.

British Library Cataloguing-in-Publication Data
A catalogue record for this book is available from the British Library

Uveitis in the Clinic - Current Approaches and Future Directions in Diagnosis, Treatment, and Patient Care
Edited by Joobin Khadamy
p. cm.
Print ISBN 978-1-83635-277-8
Online ISBN 978-1-83635-276-1
eBook (PDF) ISBN 978-1-83635-278-5

If disposing of this product, please recycle the paper responsibly.

Meet the editor

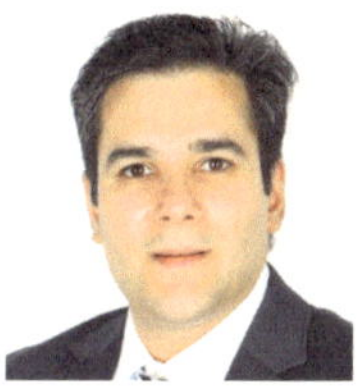

Joobin Khadamy, MD, FEBO, is a Swedish-licensed ophthalmologist and clinical researcher with expertise in cataract surgery, ocular imaging, and retinal vascular diseases. He earned his MD from Tehran University of Medical Sciences and holds the National Board of Ophthalmology from Iran. After recertifying at Umeå University in Sweden, he successfully passed the European Board of Ophthalmology (EBO) examination with distinction, earning the title of Fellow (FEBO) and receiving the Alan Ridgway Award in 2023. Dr. Khadamy has authored over 30 peer-reviewed articles, book chapters, and educational resources, and has completed hundreds of peer review assignments for international journals. He is Associate Editor for *Cureus* (Springer Nature), serves on the Reviewer Board for *Therapeutic Advances in Ophthalmology*, and is Academic Editor for *IntechOpen*. With more than 500 EyeWiki edits, he ranks among the top 20 contributors worldwide and has considerable international clinical and research experience.

Contents

Preface

Uveitis represents a diverse group of intraocular inflammatory conditions that can lead to significant visual morbidity. Its diagnosis and management require careful clinical assessment, integration of systemic findings, and, in many cases, the use of advanced diagnostic tools. This volume brings together contributions from clinicians across the world, presenting practical perspectives on both common and challenging aspects of uveitis care.

The book begins with *Diagnostic and Therapeutic Strategies in Uveitis: A Clinical Approach*, which provides a comprehensive framework for clinical evaluation, systemic work-up, and therapeutic principles. This is followed by *Anterior Segment Optical Coherence Tomography in Uveitis: Current Applications and Future Directions*, which highlights the expanding role of imaging in the assessment of inflammatory eye disease.

The second section focuses on disease-specific entities. *Tuberculous Uveitis: An Overview of Diagnosis and Management, Clinical Features and Treatment Options of Vogt–Koyanagi–Harada Disease*, and *Ocular Involvement in Behçet's Disease* provide detailed reviews of conditions that continue to present significant diagnostic and therapeutic challenges worldwide.

The final section addresses surgical and global perspectives. *Glaucoma Drainage Implants for Uveitic Glaucoma* discusses surgical approaches in complex secondary glaucoma, while *Perspective Chapter: Challenges in Managing Uveitis in Low- to Middle-Income Countries* highlights real-world barriers and adaptations in resource-limited healthcare systems.

Together, these chapters provide a structured overview of current clinical practice in uveitis, highlighting future directions in diagnosis, treatment, and research.

I want to thank the contributing authors for their commitment to this project and the editorial team for their invaluable support. I hope that this volume will serve as both a practical reference for clinicians and an academic resource for trainees and researchers interested in ocular inflammation.

Joobin Khadamy
Department of Ophthalmology,
Umeå University,
Umeå, Sweden

Section 1

Diagnostic Foundations in Uveitis

Chapter 1

Diagnostic and Therapeutic Strategies in Uveitis: A Clinical Approach

Seema Rani and Joobin Khadamy

Abstract

Uveitis refers to intraocular inflammation involving the uveal tract (iris, ciliary body, and choroid) and is a significant cause of ocular morbidity. It is responsible for a significant proportion of preventable vision loss worldwide. Uveitis can affect all age groups and often presents with eye pain, redness, photophobia, floaters, and blurred vision. It may be idiopathic or associated with systemic autoimmune diseases, infections, or trauma, and its clinical course ranges from acute to chronic. Anterior uveitis is the most common form across populations, whereas intermediate uveitis is relatively rare. Prompt diagnosis, thorough workup (including targeted laboratory tests and imaging), and appropriate therapy are critical to prevent vision-threatening complications. Management is centered on controlling inflammation with corticosteroids (topical, regional, or systemic) and immunomodulatory therapy (IMT) as needed, while addressing any underlying cause. A stepwise treatment approach is used, escalating therapy when necessary to achieve disease quiescence. Advances in ocular imaging—such as optical coherence tomography (OCT), anterior segment OCT, and fundus fluorescein angiography (FFA)—enhance diagnostic accuracy and monitoring. New therapeutic strategies, including biologic agents and intraocular drug delivery implants, have improved outcomes in refractory cases. This chapter provides an overview of uveitis classification, epidemiology, clinical evaluation, diagnostic algorithms, and evidence-based treatment strategies, illustrated by clinical cases and followed by a discussion of follow-up considerations and future directions in the management of uveitis.

Keywords: uveitis, anterior uveitis, iridocyclitis, non-granulomatous inflammation, posterior synechiae, immunomodulatory therapy, corticosteroids, OCT, HLA-B27, infectious uveitis

1. Introduction

Uveitis is an inflammation of the uvea, the pigmented middle layer of the eye lying between the sclera, the outermost layer, and retina, the innermost layer. The uveal tract consists of the iris (anterior uvea), ciliary body (intermediate uvea), and choroid (posterior uvea). Inflammation at any of these sites defines the anatomic classification of uveitis as anterior, intermediate, posterior, or panuveitis (if all segments are involved). Uveitis can be unilateral or bilateral and can affect individuals of any age. Common symptoms include eye redness, pain, light sensitivity (photophobia), floaters, and blurred vision, though the presentation can vary with the anatomic location and severity of inflammation. In anterior uveitis (iritis or iridocyclitis), patients often experience acute onset pain, redness (especially circumcorneal injection), and photophobia due to iris involvement. Intermediate uveitis (vitritis or pars planitis) and posterior uveitis (choroiditis/retinitis) may present with floaters and decreased vision, often with minimal eye redness or pain. In some chronic or pediatric cases, uveitis can be asymptomatic and detected only on routine eye examination, underscoring the importance of regular screening in at-risk groups (e.g., children with juvenile idiopathic arthritis (JIA)) [1].

Uveitis is considered an ophthalmic emergency because uncontrolled inflammation can lead to irreversible ocular damage. It accounts for about 10–15% of blindness in developed countries and roughly 30,000 new cases of legal blindness in the United States each year [2]. In up to 50% of uveitis cases, there is an associated systemic disease, most often autoimmune in nature. However, a substantial fraction remains idiopathic, despite thorough evaluation. Known *non-infectious causes* include human leukocyte antigen B27 (HLA-B27)-associated spondyloarthropathies, juvenile idiopathic arthritis (JIA), sarcoidosis, Behçet disease, Vogt-Koyanagi-Harada (VKH) syndrome, and others. *Infectious causes* encompass a range of pathogens, such as herpes simplex virus (HSV) or varicella-zoster virus (VZV) (common in anterior uveitis with keratitis), cytomegalovirus (CMV), tuberculosis, syphilis, toxoplasmosis (the most common cause of infectious posterior uveitis), toxocariasis, and others depending on geographic prevalence. Uveitic *masquerade syndromes* (conditions mimicking uveitis) like intraocular lymphoma can occur, particularly in older patients [3]. If left untreated or inadequately controlled, uveitis can result in complications including cataract, glaucoma, band keratopathy, cystoid macular edema, retinal detachment, and optic nerve damage, ultimately causing permanent vision loss.

2. Epidemiology and etiology

The epidemiology of uveitis varies by population, age, sex, and etiology. The *annual incidence* of uveitis is roughly 17 to 52 per 100,000 persons in the United States, with higher rates reported in certain regions. The *prevalence* increases with age, from approximately 30 per 100,000 in children to over 200 per 100,000 in those above 65 years. Overall, women are slightly more frequently affected than men in adult cohorts (about 57% of cases in one large study), whereas in pediatric uveitis, boys may be more often affected than girls. In 2015, an estimated 328,000 adults and 23,000 children in the United States were living with uveitis. Uveitis is broadly categorized as *non-infectious* (immune-mediated) or *infectious*, with non-infectious uveitis accounting for about 90% of cases in developed countries. In developing regions, infectious uveitis represents a larger fraction (up to 50% in some studies) due to higher prevalence of infections like tuberculosis and parasitic diseases [3, 4].

Anatomic subtype distribution: Anterior uveitis is the most common form across all ages, comprising roughly 50–80% of uveitis cases. Intermediate uveitis is less common (about 5–15% of cases) and posterior uveitis accounts for 5–30%

in different series. Panuveitis (diffuse inflammation of all segments) is the least common presentation (under 10% in most studies). Notably, more than half of intermediate uveitis cases are idiopathic (termed *pars planitis* when no systemic cause is identified). The anatomic pattern of uveitis often correlates with patient age and systemic associations. For example, pediatric uveitis is most often anterior and associated with JIA, whereas intermediate uveitis tends to present in young adults, and certain posterior uveitis entities (like birdshot chorioretinitis) are seen in middle-aged to older adults.

Age-related associations: In *children*, uveitis is relatively rare (incidence ~4 per 100,000 and prevalence ~28 per 100,000) [1], but when it occurs it is often chronic and asymptomatic. The most frequent cause of chronic anterior uveitis in children is JIA-associated uveitis [1]. JIA accounts for a large proportion of pediatric anterior uveitis in North America and Europe (from ~20 up to >60% of cases in various series) [1]. Other causes of pediatric uveitis include toxoplasmosis (a leading infectious cause of posterior uveitis in many regions) [1], toxocariasis, herpetic uveitis, and rare entities like Blau syndrome. Children more often have *idiopathic* uveitis than adults when no systemic disease is found [1]. In contrast, *young adults* (ages 20–40 years) have the highest incidence of uveitis; this group commonly presents with acute anterior uveitis, often associated with *HLA-B27* positive spondyloarthropathies (such as ankylosing spondylitis, reactive arthritis, or inflammatory bowel disease (IBD)). In fact, HLA-B27-associated disease is one of the most frequent identifiable causes of non-infectious uveitis in adults in Western countries [1]. *Middle-aged adults* may develop a wide variety of uveitis etiologies: for instance, sarcoidosis typically presents in the 30s–50s (often as granulomatous uveitis that can be anterior, intermediate, or posterior), and patients in their 40s–50s may manifest intermediate uveitis sometimes linked to multiple sclerosis (MS) or present with idiopathic posterior uveitis. *Older adults* (over 60 years) are at risk for uveitis due to viral reactivations (e.g., herpes zoster causing acute anterior uveitis with keratitis, sometimes termed *uveo-keratitis*), as well as masquerade syndromes like intraocular lymphoma [3]. Ocular sarcoidosis can also present in older adults, and intraocular lymphoma typically occurs in the elderly and must be distinguished from true inflammatory uveitis.

Sex-related associations: Females have a higher overall prevalence of uveitis than males, largely driven by autoimmune conditions (many autoimmune diseases are more common in women). Notably, juvenile idiopathic arthritis-associated uveitis predominantly affects young girls, as oligoarticular JIA is more common in females. Conversely, HLA-B27-associated acute anterior uveitis shows a male predominance, paralleling the male bias of ankylosing spondylitis and related spondyloarthropathies [5]. Behçet's disease, which can cause severe panuveitis and retinal vasculitis, is more common in men in certain populations (e.g., Middle Eastern and East Asian) [6]. Thus, patient demographics (age, sex, ethnicity) can provide important clues to the underlying cause of uveitis.

Geographic variation: The spectrum of uveitis causes varies around the world. In *developed countries*, non-infectious etiologies (e.g., HLA-B27, sarcoidosis, autoimmune uveitis) predominate. In *developing regions*, infectious uveitis is relatively more common due to higher incidence of infections like tuberculosis, leprosy, onchocerciasis, toxoplasmosis, or HIV (human immunodeficiency virus)-related ocular disease [7]. For example, tuberculosis is a leading cause of uveitis in India and parts of Africa, and ocular toxoplasmosis is a common cause of posterior uveitis in South America [1]. Even within the United States, studies have noted racial and regional differences;

for instance, sarcoid uveitis is overrepresented in Black patients in the Southeast, and certain entities like birdshot chorioretinopathy are seen almost exclusively in Caucasians. These epidemiologic patterns underscore the importance of tailoring the differential diagnosis of uveitis to the individual patient's background.

In summary, anterior uveitis is the most prevalent form of uveitis across all groups, with juvenile idiopathic arthritis serving as a key cause in children and HLA-B27-associated disease presenting as a major identifiable cause in adults [1, 5]. Posterior uveitis, though less common, is often caused by infectious agents such as *Toxoplasma gondii* (the leading cause of infectious posterior uveitis worldwide) or systemic diseases like sarcoidosis or Behçet's disease. Intermediate uveitis is frequently idiopathic but can be associated with conditions like multiple sclerosis or sarcoidosis. Overall, 30–60% of uveitis cases are considered idiopathic in many series [1], meaning no definitive cause is found, despite investigation. Given this complexity, a thoughtful approach to *etiology* is required for each uveitis patient, balancing epidemiologic likelihoods with individual clinical findings.

3. Classification of uveitis

A standardized classification helps in describing uveitis and guiding evaluation and management. The *Standardization of Uveitis Nomenclature (SUN)* Working Group [8] classifies uveitis primarily by the *anatomic site of inflammation*:

- *Anterior uveitis:* Inflammation primarily of the anterior chamber (iridocyclitis or iritis). This is the most common form of uveitis.

- *Intermediate uveitis:* Inflammation mainly in the vitreous humor and peripheral retina/pars plana (vitritis or pars planitis).

- *Posterior uveitis:* Inflammation of the retina or choroid (retinitis, choroiditis, or chorioretinitis).

- *Panuveitis:* Inflammation involving anterior chamber, vitreous, and retina/choroid simultaneously, with no single site predominating.

In addition to location, uveitis is further characterized by *onset, duration, and course*:

- *Onset: Sudden* (acute) or *insidious*. Acute uveitis often develops rapidly (within days) with pronounced symptoms, whereas insidious onset may be more gradual.

- *Duration: Limited* (acute) if it lasts <3 months or *persistent (chronic)* if it lasts ≥3 months. Acute anterior uveitis, for example, typically has a sudden onset and limited duration, while chronic uveitis (such as JIA-associated uveitis) can smolder for years.

- *Course: Acute*, *chronic*, or *recurrent*. Acute uveitis typically presents with sudden onset (<3 months). Chronic uveitis often implies persistent inflammation requiring ongoing therapy, with relapse <3 months after stopping treatment. Recurrent uveitis refers to repeated episodes separated by inactive periods ≥3 months off therapy.

Another descriptive element is the *character of inflammation*:

- *Granulomatous uveitis:* It is characterized by large "mutton-fat" keratic precipitates (KPs) on the cornea, iris nodules, and is often associated with chronic, indolent course. Granulomatous inflammation is classically seen in sarcoidosis, tuberculosis, or Vogt-Koyanagi-Harada syndrome.

- *Non-granulomatous uveitis:* Typically, it has smaller keratic precipitates, manifests as an acute onset, and is often idiopathic or associated with HLA-B27 diseases. It tends to have a brisk presentation (pain, redness), as seen in Fuchs heterochromic iridocyclitis or HLA-B27 iritis.

The SUN criteria also provide grading schemes for the level of intraocular inflammation, which are useful for standardizing assessment and monitoring response to treatment. Anterior chamber *cell and flare grading* is performed by slit-lamp examination: cells (white blood cells) are counted in a 1 × 1 mm beam and graded from 0 (none) to 4+ (>50 cells), while flare (protein in the aqueous giving haziness) is graded from 0 (none) to 4+ (intense fibrinous flare). Vitreous *cell* and *haze* are similarly graded from 0 to 4+ based on visualization of retinal details [9]. For example, a designation of "anterior uveitis, 3+ cells, 2+ flare, chronic, non-granulomatous" succinctly conveys a lot of clinical information. Precise classification is important not only for communication but also for guiding the differential diagnosis: e.g., chronic bilateral granulomatous panuveitis might prompt investigation for sarcoidosis or tuberculosis, whereas acute unilateral non-granulomatous anterior uveitis in a young adult suggests HLA-B27 etiology. Standardized diagnostic and grading systems—including the anatomic classification of uveitis (**Table 1**), SUN criteria for anterior chamber inflammation (**Tables 2** and **3**), and National Institutes of Health (NIH) grading systems for vitreous cells and haze (**Tables 4** and **5**)—are essential for accurate diagnosis, disease monitoring, and interphysician consistency.

Anatomic Type	Primary Site of Inflammation	Examples of Clinical Entities
Anterior	Anterior chamber	Non-granulomatous anterior uveitis, Fuchs uveitis, HLA-B27-associated uveitis, herpetic anterior uveitis
Intermediate	Vitreous	Pars planitis, multiple sclerosis-associated intermediate uveitis, sarcoid intermediate uveitis
Posterior	Retina or choroid	Toxoplasmosis retinochoroiditis, serpiginous choroiditis, acute retinal necrosis, cytomegalovirus retinitis
Panuveitis	Anterior chamber, vitreous, retina/choroid	Vogt-Koyanagi-Harada disease, Behçet's disease, sympathetic ophthalmia, sarcoidosis

Summarizes the Standardization of Uveitis Nomenclature (SUN) Working Group classification system, dividing uveitis into anterior, intermediate, posterior, and panuveitis, with representative clinical examples for each category.

Table 1.
Classification of uveitis by anatomic location.

Grade	Cells in the field
0	0
0.5+	1–5
1+	6–15
2+	16–25
3+	26–50
4+	50 <

Summarizes the SUN Working Group classification system with examples of typical disease entities in each category (anterior, intermediate, posterior, and panuveitis). Note that a hypopyon is not included in SUN grading and should be described separately.

Table 2.
Anterior chamber cell grading.

Grade	Cells in the field
0	No haze seen
1+	Faint haze
2+	Moderate haze with clear iris and lens details
3+	Marked inflammation with hazy visualization of the iris and lens
4+	Intense haze with fibrin or plastic aqueous seen at the slit lamp

Provides grading criteria for anterior chamber flare, as standardized by the SUN Working Group classification system.

Table 3.
Anterior chamber flare grading.

Grade	Cells in the field (1 mm X 0.5 mm)
0	No cells
0.5+	1–10
1+	10–20
2+	20–30
3+	30–100
4+	>100

Performs grading of vitreous cells using a 0.5 mm × 1 mm slit beam through the pupil, assessing the anterior vitreous. This method is used to quantify posterior segment inflammation in uveitis [9].

Table 4.
NIH grading system for vitreous cells.

Grade	Cells in the field
0	Normal findings of no haze
0.5+	Slight blurring of the optic disc margin
1+	Obscured view with definition to the optic nerve head and retinal vessels
2+	Obscured view with definition to the retinal vessels
3+	Optic nerve head is visualized, but with blurry borders
4+	Obscured fundal view

Outlines the NIH grading scale for vitreous haze, based on visibility of fundus landmarks. This is commonly used to quantify posterior segment inflammation in uveitis [9].

Table 5.
NIH grading system for vitreous haze.

4. Clinical presentation and evaluation

The clinical evaluation of uveitis involves correlating symptoms with thorough ocular examination and targeted investigations. Key steps include:

1. *History:* A detailed medical history is essential. Important aspects are onset and duration of ocular symptoms, laterality (one or both eyes), associated systemic symptoms (such as joint pain, skin rash, oral ulcers, respiratory symptoms, etc.), past medical diagnoses (autoimmune diseases, infections, malignancies), recent infections or travel, trauma or surgery, and medication use. For example, lower back stiffness might suggest ankylosing spondylitis in a patient with recurrent anterior uveitis, whereas cough or pulmonary issues could point toward sarcoidosis or tuberculosis if uveitis is granulomatous. In pediatric cases, a history of arthritis (JIA) or rash (e.g., psoriasis) is relevant. A review of systems often uncovers clues to systemic associations.

2. *Ocular examination:* A comprehensive eye examination by an ophthalmologist is mandatory. This includes the assessment of visual acuity, pupillary reactions, and intraocular pressure (IOP), followed by slit-lamp examination of the anterior segment. Slit-lamp findings in active uveitis may include conjunctival injection (especially around the cornea in ciliary flush), keratic precipitates (KPs) on the corneal endothelium (fine KP in non-granulomatous uveitis and "mutton-fat" greasy KP in granulomatous uveitis), anterior chamber cells and flare, fibrin or hypopyon (layered white cells) in severe cases, and posterior synechiae (adhesions of the iris to the lens) in prolonged inflammation. The presence of iris nodules (Busacca or Koeppe nodules) suggests granulomatous inflammation. The examiner will also check the lens (looking for cataract, which can result from inflammation or steroid therapy) and perform a funduscopic examination of the vitreous, retina, and optic disc. Posterior segment examination findings can include vitreous cells or opacities (haze), retinal lesions (e.g., yellow-white patches of retinitis, choroidal granulomas, vasculitis sheathing of retinal vessels), optic disc swelling, or hemorrhages. For intermediate uveitis, classic signs are "*snowballs*" (clumps of inflammatory cells in the vitreous) and "*snowbanking*" (inflammatory exudates over the pars plana). In posterior uveitis, one might see focal retinochoroidal scars (e.g., healed toxoplasmosis appears as a pigmented scar in the retina with adjacent active white lesion in recurrence) or widespread vascular changes in vasculitis (like periphlebitis in Eales disease or sarcoidosis).

3. *Laboratory investigations:* There is no single "uveitis panel" that fits all patients; investigations are guided by clinical suspicion. *Baseline tests* often include a complete blood count (CBC) and basic inflammatory markers (such as erythrocyte sedimentation rate (ESR) or C-reactive protein (CRP)) to check for general inflammation or hematologic abnormalities. *Infectious screenings* are of high yield: *Syphilis serology* (e.g., Rapid Plasma Reagin (RPR) or Venereal Disease Research Laboratory (VDRL) and treponemal-specific test) is recommended in *all* cases of uveitis because syphilitic uveitis is known as "the great masquerader" and can mimic any uveitis type. A *Tuberculosis* (TB) workup (Interferon Gamma Release Assay (IGRA) blood test or Purified Protein Derivative (PPD) skin test and chest X-ray or computed tomography (CT)) is indicated, especially for chronic granu-

lomatous uveitis or if the patient has risk factors for TB. A *chest X-ray* or chest CT is useful if sarcoidosis or TB is suspected, potentially revealing hilar lymphadenopathy or lung lesions. Depending on clinical clues, additional tests are pursued: for instance, *HLA-B27* testing in a patient with recurrent acute anterior uveitis (especially if male and with back pain history); *lysozyme* and *angiotensin-converting enzyme (ACE)* levels for suspected sarcoidosis (though ACE has limitations); *Lyme disease* titers in endemic areas for intermediate or posterior uveitis; and *viral serologies or polymerase chain reaction (PCR)* analysis of intraocular fluid if viral uveitis is suspected (e.g., HSV, VZV, or CMV can be confirmed via aqueous humor PCR if necrotizing retinitis or atypical anterior uveitis is present). In certain posterior uveitis cases, especially atypical or refractory ones, an *aqueous or vitreous tap* for *PCR* and even a diagnostic vitrectomy or chorioretinal biopsy might be necessary to distinguish infection from malignancy [10].

4. *Imaging:* Targeted systemic imaging studies can be very informative. A chest CT may show lung nodules or lymphadenopathy for sarcoidosis or TB. Sacroiliac joint X-rays or magnetic resonance imaging (MRI) can confirm ankylosing spondylitis in HLA-B27 uveitis patients with back pain. If intraocular lymphoma is in the differential (elderly patient with posterior uveitis unresponsive to steroids), MRI of the brain and orbits and a lumbar puncture for central nervous system (CNS) lymphoma markers may be warranted. *Ocular imaging modalities* are also invaluable in uveitis (discussed further below in *Imaging in uveitis*).

The guiding principle is to *tailor the workup* to the individual. For example, a young woman with bilateral granulomatous uveitis and lung symptoms might get ACE levels and a chest CT to evaluate for sarcoidosis, whereas an older male with unilateral anterior uveitis and high intraocular pressure should be tested for herpes virus. At the same time, some tests are broadly applied because of disease severity or treatability (as noted, syphilis and TB are routinely screened, as is COVID-19 in recent times by some protocols). **Table 1** outlines common investigations and their indications:

- *Complete blood count (CBC):* General health indicator; may show anemia (chronic disease) or abnormal white cell counts (e.g., leukemia masquerade).
- *ESR and CRP:* Non-specific inflammation markers; elevated in many systemic inflammatory conditions.
- *Syphilis serology:* Required for all uveitis patients (rules out ocular syphilis, a "masquerader").
- *Tuberculosis tests (IGRA or PPD) and chest X-ray/CT:* Indicated in chronic, granulomatous, or posterior uveitis, or if TB exposure risk; looking for evidence of TB or sarcoid in chest.
- *HLA-B27:* For recurrent acute anterior uveitis, especially if asymmetric and associated with arthritis or gastrointestinal (GI) symptoms.
- *ANA (antinuclear antibody):* In children with anterior uveitis, to evaluate JIA (young children with JIA-associated uveitis often are ANA-positive, even without overt arthritis).

DOI: http://dx.doi.org/10.5772/intechopen.1012490

- *Rheumatoid factor, cyclic citrullinated peptide (CCP) antibody:* If an adult patient has arthritis plus uveitis (though rheumatoid arthritis itself rarely causes uveitis, except secondary Sjögren's or related conditions).

- *Lyme titer:* In cases of intermediate or posterior uveitis in Lyme-endemic areas or if history suggests it.

- *Toxoplasmosis immunoglobulin G/immunoglobulin M (IgG/IgM):* For suspected toxoplasmic retinochoroiditis (though clinical diagnosis is usually sufficient).

- *Toxocara enzyme-linked immunosorbent assay (ELISA):* In children or young adults with granulomatous posterior uveitis and peripheral "snowbank"-like granulomas or a history of dog exposure (suspect ocular toxocariasis).

- *Viral PCR on aqueous fluid:* In necrotizing retinitis (to differentiate herpes simplex, varicella-zoster, or CMV retinitis) or in atypical anterior uveitis with high intraocular pressure (to detect herpetic uveitis).

- *Serologic tests for others:* e.g., *Behçet's disease* (pathergy test and HLA-B51) [6], *Vogt-Koyanagi-Harada* [11] (often clinical diagnosis; lumbar puncture shows pleocytosis), etc., as clinically indicated.

The diagnostic algorithm below (**Figure 1**) provides a structured framework guiding clinicians through clinical evaluation and targeted investigations, enhancing diagnostic accuracy in uveitis.

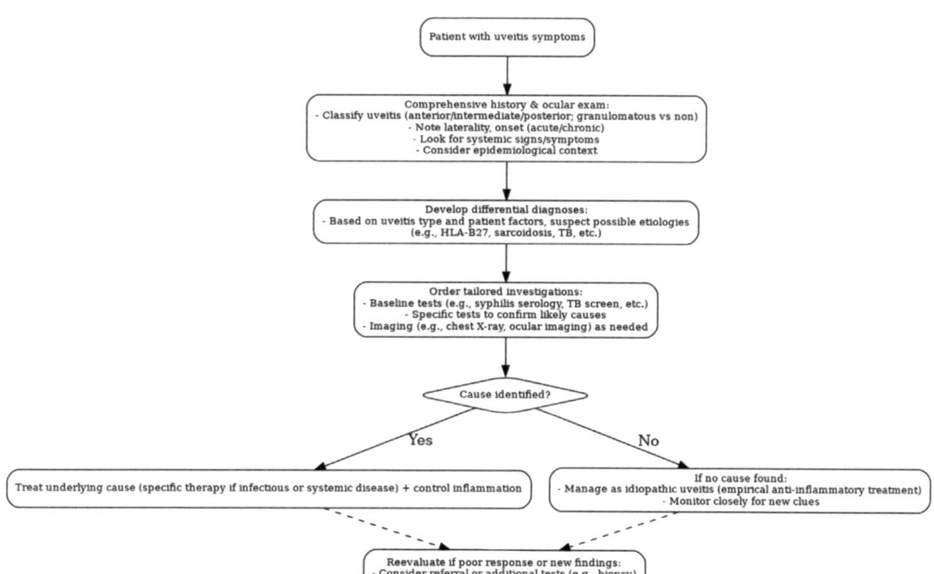

Figure 1.
Diagnostic algorithm for uveitis. This flowchart categorizes uveitis by anatomic location and key clinical features, then outlines an investigative pathway to identify common causes of uveitis. The algorithm emphasizes ruling out infections (syphilis, TB, viral, etc.), checking for systemic associations (HLA-B27 diseases, sarcoidosis, JIA, etc.), and recognizing when to consider masquerade syndromes. It provides a stepwise approach to reach a diagnosis or classify the uveitis as idiopathic after appropriate evaluation.

It must be emphasized that up to one-third of uveitis cases remain idiopathic after evaluation [5]. The clinician should avoid ordering an exhaustive battery of tests without indications; instead, a focused approach is recommended to avoid false positives and unnecessary costs. Guidelines and expert panels exist to aid in deciding which tests to order based on uveitis type [10]. For instance, one approach suggests always testing for syphilis and tuberculosis in any posterior or panuveitis, and adding tests for sarcoidosis (ACE, chest imaging) in granulomatous cases, and HLA-B27 in acute anterior cases. A close collaboration with internists, rheumatologists, or infectious disease specialists may be required to interpret results and manage systemic disease.

5. Imaging in uveitis

Advanced ophthalmic imaging techniques have become integral to the diagnosis and management of uveitis. These modalities allow for objective documentation of inflammation and detection of subtle changes that may not be obvious on clinical examination:

- *Optical coherence tomography (OCT):* Macular OCT is a non-invasive cross-sectional imaging of the retina, crucial for detecting and monitoring cystoid macular edema (CME), a common cause of vision loss in uveitis. Even mild macular thickening due to inflammation can be quantitatively monitored with OCT. OCT can also reveal epiretinal membranes or vitreomacular traction that may occur in chronic uveitis. In posterior uveitis, OCT is useful to visualize structural changes like subretinal fluid or choroidal swelling (e.g., serous retinal detachments in VKH disease). Additionally, *enhanced depth OCT* can be used to assess choroidal thickness, which may be increased in conditions like VKH or posterior scleritis. OCT is non-contact and can be done at each visit, making it ideal for following disease activity and treatment response (resolution of CME, etc.) [12, 13].

- *Anterior Segment OCT (AS-OCT):* AS-OCT is used to image the anterior eye, providing high-resolution images of the cornea, anterior chamber, iris, and angle. In uveitis, AS-OCT can objectively show anterior chamber debris or fibrin, iris adhesions, or angle closure from peripheral anterior synechiae. It is particularly useful in chronic anterior uveitis to detect subclinical inflammation or structural changes (e.g., angle closure or iris bombe). Another modality, *ultrasound biomicroscopy (UBM)*, can also be used to evaluate the anterior segment (like detecting cyclitic membranes in hypotony due to chronic uveitis), but AS-OCT is quicker and non-invasive for many anterior findings [14, 15].

- *Fundus fluorescein angiography (FFA) or fluorescein angiography (FA):* Fluorescein angiography involves intravenous injection of fluorescein dye and photographing the retinal circulation. In uveitis, FA is invaluable for assessing *retinal vasculitis* (leakage from inflamed vessels), identifying areas of non-perfusion or ischemia, detecting *cystoid macular edema* (as petaloid dye leakage in the macula), and looking for disc leakage (papillitis). For example, in intermediate uveitis or panuveitis, FA might show leakage from peripheral veins or the optic disc even if the fundus appears quiet, guiding escalation of therapy. In conditions like Behçet's disease, FA is key to monitoring retinal vasculitis severity. FA can also highlight choroidal lesions in posterior uveitis as window defects or pinpoint leaks. *Indocyanine Green Angiography (ICGA)* is another angiographic method better for choroidal circulation; it can help visualize choroidal inflammation (e.g., in birdshot chorioretinopathy or VKH) that may not be evident on FA.

- *Fundus autofluorescence (FAF):* While not asked in the prompt explicitly, FAF is sometimes employed to detect damage to the retinal pigment epithelium from chronic inflammation (e.g., in multifocal choroiditis or birdshot, lesions have characteristic autofluorescence patterns).

- *Ultrasound B-scan:* In eyes with media opacity (dense vitritis, hyphema, cataract), B-scan ultrasound can check for retinal detachment or choroidal thickening. It is also used to monitor posterior scleritis (T-sign) and to detect calcific lesions (e.g., granulomas) or tumors masquerading as uveitis.

These imaging tools greatly enhance the clinician's ability to *quantify inflammation* and *detect complications*. For instance, OCT detection of macular edema might prompt augmentation of therapy, even if the patient's vision is only slightly down [12]. Likewise, FA evidence of peripheral vasculitis could justify adding immunosuppressive treatment in an otherwise asymptomatic eye to prevent future ischemic damage. Imaging is also essential in clinical trials as objective endpoints. In practice, a combination of modalities is often used: OCT at each visit for any uveitis with potential macular involvement, and FA/ICG (Indocyanine Green) on baseline and as needed for posterior uveitis cases. AS-OCT is used in research and some clinics to follow anterior chamber inflammation objectively (quantifying anterior chamber cells) [15]. As technology progresses, *adaptive optics imaging* and *OCT angiography (OCTA)* are emerging, which may allow even more precise monitoring of inflammatory changes at the cellular or microvascular level. These advanced imaging modalities will be discussed in detail in a dedicated chapter on ocular imaging in uveitis later in this volume. For now, it is important to recognize that integrating imaging findings with clinical examination improves overall assessment and guides management decisions in uveitis care.

6. Diagnostic approach and algorithm

Uveitis requires a structured yet flexible diagnostic approach. A useful *diagnostic algorithm* involves sequential consideration of the uveitis characteristics and patient factors:

Step 1: Classify the uveitis by anatomy and onset. Determine if the case is anterior, intermediate, posterior, or panuveitis, and whether it is acute or chronic, granulomatous or non-granulomatous. This initial classification narrows down the differential diagnosis. For example, an acute unilateral anterior uveitis suggests a different set of causes (e.g., HLA-B27, Posner-Schlossman syndrome, herpetic uveitis) than a chronic bilateral granulomatous panuveitis (e.g., sarcoidosis, TB, syphilis, VKH).

Once the uveitis has been classified anatomically and key clinical characteristics have been noted (such as granulomatous vs. non-granulomatous appearance, laterality, and course), the clinician can narrow down the differential diagnosis by aligning the presentation pattern with typical underlying causes.

Table 6 provides a condensed reference to common etiologies based on anatomical subtype, onset, and other distinguishing features. This format is intended to support rapid, targeted diagnostic workup in clinical practice.

Step 2: Identify any red flags for infectious causes. Infectious uveitis must be recognized early, as treatment differs (requires antimicrobial therapy and avoids systemic immunosuppression, until infection is controlled). Clues to infection include a *necrotizing retinitis* (suggestive of viral or toxoplasmic infection), a *granulomatous anterior uveitis with high intraocular pressure* (herpetic etiology likely), or *bilateral granulomatous uveitis with choroiditis* (think tuberculosis or syphilis). If infectious uveitis is suspected, appropriate laboratory tests (e.g., syphilis, PCR of aqueous for viral DNA, toxoplasmosis titers, PPD/IGRA for TB) should be ordered promptly. In fulminant cases (like acute retinal necrosis), one might even treat empirically for the infection while awaiting results. Aqueous or vitreous sampling for PCR can confirm diagnoses like viral retinitis or ocular toxoplasmosis. Always *rule out syphilis and tuberculosis* in any atypical or severe uveitis, as these are treatable causes not to miss [5].

Step 3: Assess for systemic disease association. This involves a thorough review of systems and possibly rheumatologic evaluation. For non-infectious uveitis, consider:

Clinical pattern/ presentation	Possible etiologies
Anterior uveitis	Non-specific/idiopathic; HLA-B27-associated spondyloarthropathies (ankylosing spondylitis, inflammatory bowel disease, psoriatic arthritis, reactive arthritis); sarcoidosis; juvenile idiopathic arthritis (JIA); tubulointerstitial nephritis with uveitis (TINU); lens-related inflammation; Posner-Schlossman syndrome; Fuchs uveitis; Lyme borreliosis; herpetic viruses (HSV, VZV, CMV); tuberculosis; syphilis.
Intermediate uveitis	Pars planitis (idiopathic); sarcoidosis; inflammatory bowel disease; multiple sclerosis; Lyme borreliosis.
Posterior uveitis	Idiopathic; toxoplasmosis; sarcoidosis; tuberculosis; syphilis; fungal infections (e.g., *Candida,Histoplasma*); viral retinitides (acute retinal necrosis, progressive outer retinal necrosis, CMV retinitis); intraocular lymphoma; white-dot syndromes.
Bilateral uveitis	Idiopathic; sarcoidosis; JIA; TINU; tuberculosis; syphilis; Lyme borreliosis; Behçet's disease.
Granulomatous uveitis	Idiopathic; herpetic viruses; toxoplasmosis; tuberculosis; syphilis; Lyme borreliosis; sarcoidosis; Posner-Schlossman syndrome; chronic low-grade inflammation (e.g., Fuchs uveitis).
Uveitis with elevated intraocular pressure	Posner-Schlossman syndrome; Schwartz-Matsuo syndrome; sarcoidosis; toxoplasmosis; herpetic uveitis.
Slow, insidious onset	Idiopathic; JIA; Fuchs uveitis; sarcoidosis.
Pediatric presentations	JIA (often more frequent than idiopathic); idiopathic; pars planitis; post-viral neuroretinitis; ocular toxocariasis; TINU.
Panuveitis	Idiopathic; sarcoidosis; Behçet's disease; sympathetic ophthalmia; Vogt-Koyanagi-Harada (VKH) disease.
Hypopyon	Infective endophthalmitis; HLA-B27 associated entities (ankylosing spondylitis, IBD, reactive arthritis); Behçet's disease.
Conditions with high risk of rapid or severe vision loss	*Rapid onset*: Acute retinal necrosis, Behçet's disease. *Slow progression*: ocular tuberculosis, sarcoidosis.

Table 6.
Pattern-based differential diagnoses in uveitis.

DOI: http://dx.doi.org/10.5772/intechopen.1012490

- *HLA-B27-associated disease:* Usually acute, unilateral (alternating) anterior uveitis in a patient (often male) with a history of back pain, arthritis, psoriasis, or inflammatory bowel disease. Test HLA-B27; if positive, refer to a rheumatologist for evaluation of spondyloarthritis.

- *Sarcoidosis:* Often chronic, granulomatous uveitis (anterior, intermediate, or posterior). Look for systemic signs (pulmonary, cutaneous, etc.). Order ACE level, chest imaging. *Elevated ACE or chest lymphadenopathy* supports the diagnosis, though biopsy (of accessible lymph nodes or lung) is the gold standard for confirmation.

- *Juvenile idiopathic arthritis (JIA):* In any child or adolescent with chronic anterior uveitis, especially if ANA-positive young girl, consider JIA even if joint symptoms are minimal. In known JIA patients, regular screening eye examinations are crucial since their uveitis can be asymptomatic.

- *Behçet's disease:* Panuveitis with retinal vasculitis in a young adult (often male) with oral and genital ulcers is suggestive. Pathergy test and HLA-B51 may aid diagnosis. Behçet's requires prompt systemic immunosuppression to prevent severe vision loss from occlusive vasculitis.

- *Vogt-Koyanagi-Harada (VKH) syndrome:* Consider diffuse bilateral granulomatous uveitis in a middle-aged patient, often with prodromal meningitic symptoms, skin or hair depigmentation (poliosis, vitiligo), or hearing loss. VKH commonly presents with bilateral exudative retinal detachments (seen on examination or OCT) and requires aggressive systemic corticosteroids.

- *Multiple sclerosis (MS):* Intermediate uveitis (pars planitis) in adults, especially if bilateral and accompanied by neurologic symptoms (optic neuritis history, numbness, etc.), may be associated with MS. Brain MRI is indicated if MS is suspected, as about 20% of intermediate uveitis cases have or will develop MS [16].

- *Masquerade syndromes:* If the clinical picture is unusual (e.g., uveitis not responding to steroids or presence of malignant cells in aqueous humor on cytology), consider intraocular lymphoma (primary vitreoretinal lymphoma) or leukemia. Elderly patients with new-onset "uveitis" should raise suspicion for masquerade; diagnostic vitrectomy for cytology can confirm lymphoma.

Step 4: Order targeted investigations. Based on the suspected differentials from Steps 2 and 3, order the laboratory and imaging tests, as outlined in the Clinical Evaluation section. One practical algorithm is:

- *All patients:* Syphilis serology, basic inflammation markers, and chest X-ray (the latter to pick up TB or sarcoid signs).

- *If granulomatous or intermediate or multifocal choroiditis:* Add ACE level, chest CT, and TB testing (IGRA).

- *If non-granulomatous anterior uveitis in young adult:* HLA-B27, and if female child, ANA (for JIA risk).

- *If necrotizing retinitis:* Aqueous/vitreous PCR for HSV, VZV, CMV, toxoplasmosis; also syphilis and TB as these can cause posterior placoid lesions or panuveitis.

- *If vasculitis on FA:* Consider testing for Behçet's (clinical criteria), sarcoidosis, TB, and syphilis.

- *If we suspect MS:* MRI brain/spine.

- *If we suspect lymphoma:* Vitreous biopsy.

- In cases of *keratouveitis* (especially with corneal infiltrates, endothelial plaques, or hypopyon) where infection is suspected, *an anterior chamber paracentesis (AC tap)* may be performed. AC fluid can be analyzed by *PCR* (for HSV, VZV, CMV) and *culture/stain* (for bacteria, fungi, atypical organisms like TB). Early AC tap allows targeted antimicrobial therapy and avoids inappropriate steroid monotherapy.

  AC tap is especially recommended *before escalating steroids* if infectious etiology is uncertain.

By this stepwise approach, the physician can usually identify an underlying cause in a significant subset of patients or confidently treat the uveitis as idiopathic after reasonable exclusion of known causes.

Step 5: Reassess and refine diagnosis during follow-up. It is not uncommon that initial tests are negative and a patient is labeled "idiopathic." However, uveitis may be the first manifestation of a latent systemic disease. Thus, patients need ongoing monitoring for new signs or symptoms. For example, sarcoidosis might declare itself months later with a chest CT change or skin lesion that can be biopsied. Or a patient initially idiopathic may develop arthritis later, revising the diagnosis to HLA-B27 disease. The diagnostic algorithm is iterative: if a uveitis case is refractory to treatment or atypical in course, revisit the differential, repeat certain tests, or obtain second opinions. A multidisciplinary approach (involving rheumatology, infectious disease, pulmonology, etc.) maximizes the chances of securing a diagnosis.

To summarize, the diagnostic algorithm for uveitis starts with anatomic classification and identifying patterns that suggest particular etiologies, followed by judicious testing. Always exclude infectious causes early, consider systemic associations, and use laboratories/imaging in a targeted manner. **Figure 1** illustrates a simplified flow: first determine location (anterior vs. intermediate vs. posterior), then check for defining features (granulomatous? acute vs. chronic? unilateral vs. bilateral?), from which branch into likely diagnoses, and corresponding tests. If all investigations are negative, manage as idiopathic but keep the patient under surveillance for clues to emerge. This structured approach ensures efficient use of resources and timely diagnosis, which is critical for guiding therapy.

Figure 1 is a diagnostic algorithm outlining the categorization and workup of uveitis. It guides the clinician from initial anatomic classification through targeted differential diagnosis and investigations.

7. Treatment and management

The primary goal of uveitis treatment is to suppress intraocular inflammation as swiftly as possible to prevent tissue damage, while minimizing treatment side effects.

Management strategies must be tailored to the *cause, severity, and chronicity* of uveitis in each patient. Broadly, therapies include *corticosteroids*, *immunosuppressive/immunomodulatory agents*, and *surgery* when indicated, in addition to treating any underlying infection or systemic disease.

7.1 Corticosteroid therapy (first-line)

Corticosteroids are the mainstay for acute inflammation control. They can be delivered topically, regionally (injections or implants), or systemically:

- *Topical steroids:* High-potency topical corticosteroid eye drops (e.g., prednisolone acetate 1% or difluprednate 0.05%) are the first-line treatment for anterior uveitis. A typical regimen for moderate anterior uveitis might be one drop every 1–2 hours initially, then tapering as inflammation improves. Topical steroids primarily act on the anterior segment, so they are less useful for intermediate or posterior uveitis, except as adjuncts (they do not reach the back in high concentration). Topical steroids are effective in many cases of anterior uveitis, inducing remission within days to weeks. *Cycloplegic* drops (such as atropine or cyclopentolate) are often added to relieve pain from ciliary spasm and to prevent synechiae by keeping the pupil dilated.

- *Periocular steroid injections:* For intermediate uveitis, posterior uveitis, or cystoid macular edema, a local steroid injection can be very effective. A common approach is an injection of triamcinolone acetonide (40 mg) in the posterior sub-Tenon's space or orbital floor (transseptal) [17, 18]. This delivers high concentrations of steroid to the posterior segment without as much systemic absorption. Indications for periocular injection include unilateral intermediate/posterior uveitis or when local therapy is preferred over systemic (e.g., the patient cannot tolerate systemic steroids) [17]. Intravitreal steroid injections are also used, particularly the *dexamethasone intravitreal implant (Ozurdex)*, which provides sustained release for about 3–4 months, or *triamcinolone acetonide* (injectable suspension), which has a shorter-term effect. These are beneficial in severe posterior inflammation or macular edema. Risks of local steroid injections include cataract, elevated intraocular pressure (glaucoma), and in rare cases injection-related complications (infection, hemorrhage) [17].

- *Oral (systemic) steroids:* Prednisone (or equivalent) by mouth is used when inflammation is severe, sight-threatening, or not confined to the front of the eye. For example, panuveitis or posterior uveitis often requires systemic steroids to rapidly quell inflammation. A typical starting dose in adults is prednisone 40–60 mg daily (or about 1 mg/kg) [19], continued for a few weeks then tapered. Intravenous (IV) pulse steroids (e.g., methylprednisolone 500–1000 mg IV daily for 3 days) are reserved for extreme cases such as bilateral posterior uveitis with retinal detachment (as in VKH) or severe optic neuritis in Behçet's, where immediate high-dose therapy is needed. Systemic steroids have significant side effects (hyperglycemia, hypertension, osteoporosis, etc.), so they are used for the shortest duration necessary.

Under the "treat-and-taper" regimen, the aim is to control inflammation and then taper steroids to the lowest effective dose or discontinue. However, many cases of non-infectious uveitis are *chronic or recurrent*, meaning they will flare up as steroids taper off. Long-term reliance on corticosteroids is undesirable due to ocular side effects (cataracts, glaucoma) and systemic effects (if using oral steroids). Therefore, guidelines advocate for introducing *steroid-sparing immunomodulatory therapy* if the uveitis cannot be controlled with an acceptable maintenance dose of steroids. A commonly cited rule is: if a patient requires >2 topical prednisolone drops per day for >3 months, and/or systemic prednisone >7.5–10 mg/day for >3 months, then a steroid-sparing agent should be added [17]. In other words, the goal is to taper prednisone to 7.5 mg or less (a relatively safe maintenance dose) within 3–6 months [20]. If this is not achievable (inflammation flares on lower doses), then additional immunosuppressants are indicated. This strategy prevents the patient from accumulating steroid damage over time [20].

7.2 Immunomodulatory therapy (steroid-sparing treatment)

Immunomodulatory therapy (IMT) refers to non-corticosteroid systemic treatments that suppress the immune system. These are used in chronic, non-infectious uveitis to maintain remission with less reliance on steroids, following the principle of "*steroid-sparing*" management [17]. IMT is typically started and managed in collaboration with a uveitis specialist or rheumatologist. The choice of agent depends on disease severity, patient factors, and underlying systemic disease:

- *Conventional immunosuppressants:* These include antimetabolites like *methotrexate*, *mycophenolate mofetil*, and *azathioprine*; T-cell inhibitors like *cyclosporine* or *tacrolimus*; and alkylating agents like *cyclophosphamide* or *chlorambucil* (the latter reserved for severe, refractory cases, given their toxicity) [17, 21]. Methotrexate (7.5–25 mg weekly) is commonly used, especially in JIA-associated uveitis and other chronic anterior uveitis, with good efficacy and relatively well-known safety profile [22]. Mycophenolate is often chosen for intermediate or posterior uveitis and is popular due to its tolerability. Azathioprine is an older drug used in some posterior uveitis or birdshot retinochoroidopathy. Cyclosporine and tacrolimus are calcineurin inhibitors effective in intermediate and posterior uveitis, including Birdshot and VKH. These drugs can be used in combination (e.g., methotrexate + adalimumab in JIA uveitis) for synergistic effect. Treatment response may take 6–8 weeks or more, so overlap with corticosteroids is common initially. Monitoring for side effects (liver and kidney function, blood counts) is necessary.

- *Biologic agents:* Biologics have revolutionized uveitis therapy in the past decade, particularly for severe posterior uveitis and panuveitis. The prototypical biologic in uveitis is *adalimumab*, a monoclonal antibody against tumor necrosis factor alpha (TNF-α). Adalimumab has Food and Drug Administration (FDA) approval for non-infectious uveitis and has shown efficacy in controlling inflammation and reducing relapse in pivotal trials. It is given as a subcutaneous (SC) injection (usually 40 mg every 2 weeks). Other anti-TNF agents like *infliximab* (IV infusion) are also used, especially in Behçet's disease where infliximab can be highly effective. It is noted that *etanercept* (a TNF receptor fusion protein) is less effective for uveitis and even associated with new onset uveitis in some cases, so it is not generally used for treating uveitis [17]. Beyond TNF inhibitors, newer biologics target other pathways: *interleukin-6 (IL-6) inhibitor (tocilizumab)* has been used for uveitic macular edema (UME) (especially in juvenile uveitic CME) [17], and *interferon alpha (IFN-α)* has shown efficacy in Behçet's uveitis in some studies [17]. *Anti-CD20 (cluster of differentiation 20) therapy (rituximab)* has been tried in severe refractory cases or for lymphoma masquerades. The choice of biologic often depends on underlying disease: for example, TNF blockers are first-line treatment for Behçet's and useful in many idiopathic cases; if the patient has concurrent juvenile arthritis or refractory macular edema, tocilizumab might be chosen. Biologics have their own side effect profiles (risk of infection, reactivation of latent TB, demyelination, etc.) and are of high cost, so their use is typically reserved for cases that fail conventional IMT or when conventional drugs are contraindicated [17, 21].

When to initiate IMT? According to expert recommendations, IMT should be started if uveitis is vision-threatening, bilateral, or chronic enough that steroid monotherapy is inadequate or causes dependency [20]. For instance, JIA-associated uveitis almost always needs an immunosuppressive agent (methotrexate +/− biologic) because it is chronic and can lead to blindness if not aggressively managed. Similarly, a patient with panuveitis who cannot taper below prednisone 15 mg without relapse should be started on a steroid-sparing agent rather than keeping them on moderate-dose prednisone indefinitely [20]. The *Fundamentals of Care for Uveitis (FOCUS)* initiative provides guidance on use of IMT and biologics in non-infectious uveitis [23]. They emphasize early introduction of IMT for severe cases and a multidisciplinary approach. It is also worth noting that certain uveitic syndromes have specific preferred treatments: e.g., Behçet's disease often warrants early biologic therapy (infliximab or adalimumab) given the risk of rapid vision loss, whereas ocular sarcoidosis might respond to methotrexate or azathioprine.

A variety of immunosuppressive therapies are used in non-infectious uveitis, ranging from conventional agents such as methotrexate and mycophenolate (**Table 7**) to targeted biologics including TNF-α and IL-6 inhibitors for refractory or systemic disease (**Table 8**).

The therapeutic management algorithm (**Figure 2**) summarizes the stepwise escalation of treatment modalities, tailored according to severity, chronicity, and response to initial therapies.

7.3 Adjunctive therapies and surgery

In addition to anti-inflammatory medications, other therapies may be needed:

- *Antimicrobial therapy:* If an infectious cause is identified, appropriate antimicrobial treatment is paramount. Examples: ocular toxoplasmosis is treated with antimicrobials like pyrimethamine, sulfadiazine, and folinic acid (or trimethoprim-sulfamethoxazole), typically combined with systemic steroids once therapy is started. Herpetic uveitis requires systemic antivirals (e.g., acyclovir for HSV or VZV) along with topical steroids for inflammation. Tuberculous uveitis is managed with full anti-TB therapy; syphilitic uveitis with IV penicillin, etc. In these cases, corticosteroids are used only in conjunction with appropriate anti-infectives and never as sole therapy.

- *Mydriatics:* Cycloplegic drops (atropine, scopolamine, cyclopentolate) are used in anterior uveitis to relieve pain and prevent posterior synechiae by keeping the

Drug	Drug Class/Mechanism	Route	Typical Dose	Common Indications in Uveitis	Notable Adverse Effects
Methotrexate	Antimetabolite (dihydrofolate reductase inhibitor)	Oral/ Subcutaneous	7.5–25 mg weekly	Anterior uveitis, JIA-associated uveitis	Hepatotoxicity, bone marrow suppression, GI upset
Mycophenolate mofetil	Purine synthesis inhibitor	Oral	1–1.5 g twice daily	Posterior uveitis, panuveitis	GI intolerance, leukopenia, infections
Azathioprine	Purine analog/antimetabolite	Oral	1–2 mg/kg/day	Panuveitis, VKH, Behçet's disease	Bone marrow suppression, liver dysfunction
Cyclosporine	Calcineurin inhibitor	Oral	2–5 mg/kg/day	Intermediate/posterior uveitis, Behçet's	Nephrotoxicity, hypertension, hirsutism
Tacrolimus	Calcineurin inhibitor	Oral	0.1–0.2 mg/ kg/day	Refractory uveitis	Nephrotoxicity, tremor, hyperglycemia
Cyclophosphamide	Alkylating agent	Oral/IV	1–2 mg/kg/day (oral)	Severe panuveitis, systemic lupus erythematosus (SLE)-associated retinitis	Hemorrhagic cystitis, infertility, malignancy
Chlorambucil	Alkylating agent	Oral	0.1–0.2 mg/ kg/day	Behçet's disease, serpiginous choroiditis	Bone marrow suppression, malignancy risk

Lists frequently used systemic immunosuppressive agents for non-infectious uveitis, including their drug class, mechanism of action, common dosing protocols, and notable adverse effects.

Table 7.
Common immunomodulatory agents used in uveitis.

Drug Name	Target/Mechanism	Route of Administration	Indications in Uveitis	Common Adverse Effects
Adalimumab	TNF-α inhibitor	Subcutaneous injection	Non-infectious posterior or panuveitis	Injection site reactions, infections
Infliximab	TNF-α inhibitor	Intravenous infusion	Behçet's disease, VKH, refractory uveitis	Infusion reactions, increased infection risk
Tocilizumab	IL-6 receptor inhibitor	Intravenous or subcutaneous	JIA-associated uveitis, refractory CME	Neutropenia, elevated liver enzymes
Rituximab	Anti-CD20 monoclonal antibody	Intravenous infusion	Scleritis, refractory panuveitis	Infusion reaction, B-cell depletion
Abatacept	Cytotoxic T lymphocyte-associated antigen 4 immunoglobulin (CTLA-4 Ig) fusion protein	Intravenous or subcutaneous	JIA-associated uveitis	Headache, infections

Summarizes biologic immunomodulatory therapies targeting cytokines or immune cells, used in the management of non-infectious uveitis. It includes mechanisms of action, route of administration, typical clinical indications, and notable adverse effects.

Table 8.
Biologic agents commonly used in the treatment of non-infectious uveitis.

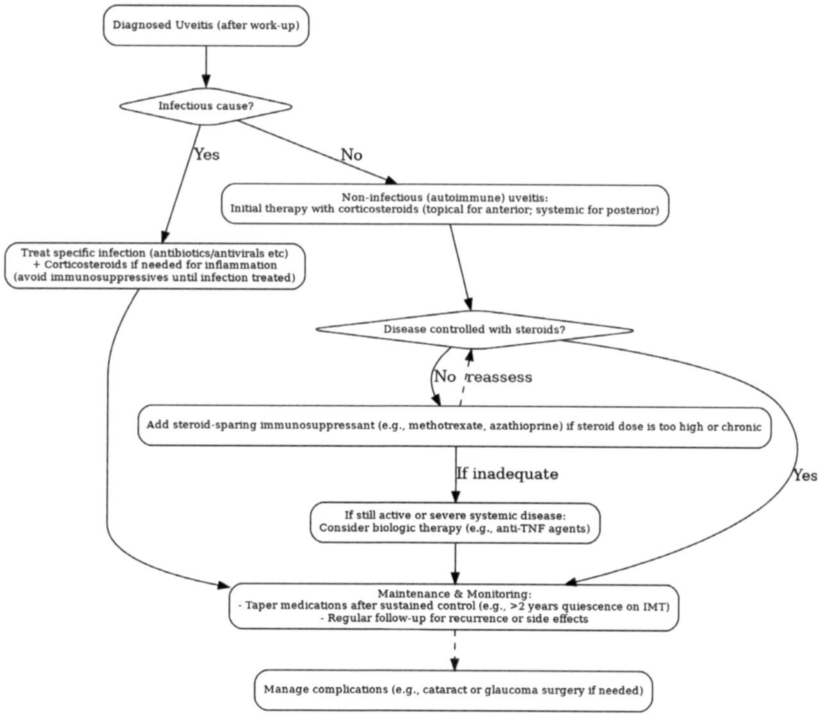

Figure 2.
Therapeutic approach to uveitis based on disease severity and response. The algorithm outlines escalation from corticosteroids to systemic immunosuppressants and biologics, with adjunctive treatments and indications for surgical intervention.

pupil dilated and the iris mobile. They are an important supportive treatment in acute iridocyclitis.

- *Intraocular pressure lowering:* Uveitis and corticosteroids can both elevate intraocular pressure (IOP). Topical glaucoma medications (like beta-blockers, carbonic anhydrase inhibitors) may be needed to control IOP. Prostaglandin analogs are relatively contraindicated as they might exacerbate inflammation. If IOP remains uncontrolled (chronic uveitic glaucoma), surgical intervention such as glaucoma drainage implant may be required [24].

- *Surgical intervention:* While medical therapy is the mainstay, surgery is indicated in certain scenarios. *Cataract surgery* is often needed in uveitis patients because long-term inflammation and steroid use commonly lead to cataract formation. Cataract surgery in uveitic eyes should be done when inflammation is quiescent (at least 3 months of control) to reduce postoperative flares. *Vitrectomy* can be both diagnostic and therapeutic: removing vitreous can help treat intermediate uveitis with non-resolving vitreous haze or floaters, and also allows for diagnostic sampling. In cases of *vitreomacular traction or epiretinal membranes* from chronic inflammation, vitrectomy with membrane peeling can improve vision. Posterior uveitis may predispose to retinal tears or detachments due to chronic vitreoretinal traction. *Retinal detachment repair* may be needed if uveitis led to tears or exudative detachment [25]. In specific diseases like JIA-associated uveitis, aggressive complications (band keratopathy, glaucoma, cataract) often mean multiple surgeries over a patient's lifetime. Another surgical modality is *intravitreal steroid implants*: the Retisert (fluocinolone acetonide implant) is a surgically placed implant that delivers steroid to the eye for up to 30 months and is FDA-approved for chronic non-infectious posterior uveitis. It is very effective at controlling inflammation but nearly always causes cataract and often glaucoma requiring surgical management. The newer Yutiq implant (fluocinolone 36-month injectable) and Ozurdex (dexamethasone 3-month injectable) provide options for long-term local steroid delivery. The decision to use these implants is made if systemic therapy is not possible or not sufficient and the disease is unilateral or asymmetric. Additionally, *laser photocoagulation* might be used adjunctively in cases of ischemic retinal vasculitis to prevent neovascularization.

7.3.1 Monitoring and adjusting treatment

Uveitis treatment is a dynamic process. Patients are seen frequently during active phases (every 1–2 weeks for severe anterior uveitis, for example) and the treatment is adjusted based on response. The SUN criteria grading is used to quantify improvement (e.g., anterior chamber cells decreasing from 3+ to 1+ after 2 weeks of prednisone). Once inflammation is quiet (zero cells), the maintenance phase involves tapering steroids to find the minimum required dose and continuing immunosuppressants for a long enough duration (often at least 1–2 years of quiescence before considering taper of IMT). Therapy must also be adjusted for side effects—if a patient develops high IOP from steroids, one may switch from drops to systemic or to a steroid-sparing agent faster. Patients on systemic IMT require blood test monitoring (for liver enzymes, blood counts, etc.) and those on biologics need screening for infections (TB, hepatitis B) prior to initiation.

In summary, the treatment of uveitis begins with corticosteroids to quickly control inflammation, but long-term management hinges on immunomodulatory therapy in many cases to avoid steroid overuse. The approach is stepwise: start local treatment for mild unilateral cases, systemic treatment for bilateral or severe cases, and escalate to immunosuppressives or biologics if steroid-sparing is needed [17]. Throughout, treat any underlying cause (infection or systemic disease) in parallel. The adage is "treat the patient, not just the eye"—meaning systemic associations must be managed (e.g., rheumatologic therapy for ankylosing spondylitis, antibiotics for TB) in order to truly control the uveitis and prevent recurrences.

7.4 Special situations: Uveitis and pregnancy

During pregnancy, several hormonal and immunological changes alter the immune response, which can affect the course of uveitis. Disease activity tends to *flare more frequently during the first trimester*, followed by *improvement during the second and third trimesters*, likely due to increased immunotolerance. However, a significant risk of *relapse exists postpartum*, requiring close follow-up after delivery.

Management of non-infectious uveitis during pregnancy necessitates a *multidisciplinary approach*, involving the ophthalmologist, obstetrician, and often a rheumatologist. The primary goal is to *minimize fetal risk while maintaining maternal disease control*.

- *First-line treatment* involves the *lowest effective dose of corticosteroids*, with a preference for *local therapies* (topical, periocular injections) to reduce systemic exposure.

- If systemic therapy becomes necessary, *corticosteroids* (e.g., oral prednisone at the lowest effective dose) can be used cautiously, as they are relatively safe during pregnancy.

- In cases requiring steroid-sparing immunomodulatory therapy, agents such as *Cyclosporine*, *Azathioprine*, and *Certolizumab pegol* (a PEGylated anti-TNF agent lacking fragment crystallizable (FC) region for placental transfer [26] are considered relatively safe based on current data.

- *Methotrexate*, *Mycophenolate Mofetil*, and *Cyclophosphamide* are *contraindicated* in pregnancy due to teratogenicity and should be discontinued prior to conception.

A close monitoring of uveitis activity is essential throughout pregnancy, with adjustment of therapies based on disease control. Proactive planning is also recommended for women of reproductive age receiving teratogenic agents, including *contraceptive counseling* and *pre-conception medication adjustments,* when necessary [27].

8. Follow-up and prognosis

Uveitis requires careful follow-up due to its often prolonged course and risk of recurrence. Follow-up strategies depend on the uveitis type and severity:

- *Acute anterior uveitis:* Patients are typically seen 1–2 weeks after initiating therapy. If improving, follow-up can be every 2 weeks until the anterior chamber is quiet and the steroid drops are tapered to a low frequency. Once quiescent, the patient may be monitored every 1–3 months for relapse. They should be educated on recognizing early symptoms of flare (redness, photophobia) and to return promptly if these occur. Prognosis for idiopathic or HLA-B27 anterior uveitis is generally good if treated early, but recurrence is common (many HLA-B27 patients have repeat attacks). Each recurrence is treated similarly, and some patients with frequent flares benefit from maintenance nonsteroidal anti-inflammatory drugs (NSAIDs) or immunosuppressants to reduce relapses.

- *Chronic anterior uveitis (e.g., JIA-associated):* These patients need very close monitoring, often every 4–6 weeks even when quiet, because smoldering inflammation can cause damage without obvious symptoms. In pediatric uveitis, complications like band keratopathy or glaucoma can develop insidiously. Regular examinations (with careful slit-lamp and pressure checks) are essential. Screening guidelines for JIA uveitis recommend eye examinations every 3 to 12 months depending on the risk category (ANA status, age at JIA onset, disease duration). Prognosis in chronic uveitis is guarded—long-term outcomes depend on maintaining control of inflammation. With modern immunosuppressive therapy (e.g., biologics), outcomes have improved, and many children retain functional vision into adulthood if managed aggressively [28]. However, chronic uveitis still carries significant risk of cataracts, glaucoma, and vision loss if not well controlled.

- *Intermediate uveitis:* Even though intermediate uveitis often has a mild course subjectively, it can quietly cause macular edema and vision loss. Follow-up every 2–3 months is typical if the disease is stable, with OCT at each visit to check the macula. If on therapy (e.g., methotrexate), visits are scheduled to coincide with laboratory monitoring. Prognosis varies—pars planitis can burn out after some years or persist. A significant number (up to one-third) of intermediate uveitis patients may ultimately develop complications like CME or retinal detachment that threaten vision [16]. With therapy (steroids, anti-VEGF (vascular endothelial growth factor) for edema, etc.), many can maintain good vision for years.

- *Posterior uveitis and panuveitis:* These are the most vision-threatening and thus require frequent follow-ups. Active retinal inflammation may need weekly or biweekly checks initially. As things improve, follow-ups are spaced to monthly. Patients on systemic immunosuppressives need regular systemic monitoring as well (blood tests usually every 4–8 weeks). Because posterior uveitis often flares unpredictably, long-term (multiyear) therapy is common. For example, a patient with birdshot chorioretinopathy may be on cyclosporine and mycophenolate for 3–5 years and followed monthly to bimonthly, using FA periodically to ensure no recurrence of vasculitis. Even after tapering off medications, such patients need intermittent follow-up (e.g., every 6 months) as relapses can occur after years of remission. Prognosis in posterior uveitis depends on the cause: entities like birdshot or VKH can often be controlled with immunosuppression, whereas Behçet's disease can be aggressive but biologics have improved its outlook significantly. Infectious posterior uveitis like toxoplasmosis has a good prognosis if treated early, though recurrences can happen and each episode can cumulatively damage the retina.

Follow-up visits always include looking for complications: *cataract* (any persistent steroid use or chronic inflammation will eventually cause lens opacities), *glaucoma* (check IOP every visit, as uveitic glaucoma is a leading cause of permanent vision loss), *macular edema* (OCT each visit if macula was ever involved), and *secondary membrane formation* (such as cyclitic membranes causing hypotony). If complications are identified, they are addressed promptly—e.g., cataract surgery when indicated, glaucoma filtering surgery if medications are not enough, Ozurdex implant for recalcitrant macular edema, etc.

Patient education is a vital component of follow-up. Patients should understand the chronic nature of many uveitis conditions and the importance of medication adherence. They should also be counseled about medication side effects (e.g., get bone protection and regular DEXA (dual-energy X-ray absorptiometry) scans if on long-term steroids, have blood sugar monitored, etc.). Those on immunosuppressants should be educated on infection precautions and the need for regular laboratory tests.

Prognosis: With appropriate therapy, many patients with uveitis can maintain good vision in at least one eye. Historically, uveitis carried a poor prognosis—studies from tertiary centers in the 1990s showed up to 25% of uveitis patients becoming legally blind in at least one eye. Modern treatment has improved these outcomes, especially due to earlier use of immunosuppressives and biologics that control inflammation more effectively. Nevertheless, certain diagnoses still have guarded prognoses (e.g., sympathetic ophthalmia or extensive posterior segment destruction). Key prognostic factors include the *duration of active inflammation* (the longer the eye stays inflamed, the worse the outcome), the *presence of structural complications* at presentation (e.g., chronic macular edema or optic atrophy portends worse vision), and *response to therapy*. Rapid control of inflammation and careful prevention of recurrences give the best chance for visual preservation. Multidisciplinary care improves outcomes in systemic cases—e.g., a rheumatologist co-managing JIA or sarcoidosis ensures systemic disease is adequately treated alongside the ocular disease. In summary, while uveitis remains a potentially blinding group of diseases, timely and aggressive management coupled with vigilant follow-up can result in favorable outcomes for the majority of patients.

9. Clinical cases

To illustrate the principles of diagnosis and management, four clinical cases are presented below:

Case 1—HLA-B27-associated acute anterior uveitis: A 28-year-old man presents with a sudden onset of pain, redness, and photophobia in his right eye for 3 days. He notes a history of similar episodes in the past affecting either eye, which improved with some steroid eye drops. He also reports chronic lower back pain and morning stiffness that improves with exercise. On examination, visual acuity is 20/25 in the right eye and 20/20 in the left eye. The right eye shows ciliary injection, 3+ anterior chamber cells and 2+ flare, and a few fine keratic precipitates on the cornea. The pupil is slightly irregular due to posterior synechiae. Intraocular pressure is 18 mmHg OD (right eye) and 12 mmHg OS (left eye). The left eye is quiet. No vitreous cells or fundus lesions are seen in either eye. This presentation is consistent with *recurrent acute anterior uveitis*, likely due to an HLA-B27-associated spondyloarthropathy (given the bilateral alternating nature and back pain). Workup was notable for HLA-B27 positivity; MRI of the sacroiliac joints showed sacroiliitis confirming ankylosing spondylitis

[29]. Syphilis and TB tests were negative. The patient was treated with aggressive topical corticosteroids (prednisolone acetate 1% hourly) and cycloplegic (atropine 1% once daily). Within 1 week, the pain resolved and inflammation reduced to 1+ cells. A slow taper of steroids was done over 6 weeks. He was referred to a rheumatologist for management of ankylosing spondylitis and started on NSAIDs. Over the next year, he had two more flares of uveitis, at which point *methotrexate* was initiated to reduce recurrences. At last follow-up (2 years after initial visit), he is maintained on low-dose methotrexate and has been flare-free for 12 months with 20/20 vision each eye. *Discussion:* This case demonstrates a classic anterior uveitis associated with a systemic disease. Prompt use of topical steroids led to quick remission. The recurrence pattern and need for prolonged treatment justified immunomodulatory therapy to prevent cumulative damage. It also highlights the importance of systemic evaluation: identification of ankylosing spondylitis allowed appropriate specialist care and improved overall outcomes. With coordinated care, the patient's ocular and systemic conditions are well controlled. This case also emphasizes that HLA-B27 uveitis often alternates eyes and can lead to posterior synechiae—hence, the use of cycloplegics. Prognosis in such cases is excellent if flares are treated early and long-term strategies (like immunosuppression or biologics) are employed for frequent relapses.

Case 2—Tuberculous granulomatous uveitis: A 45-year-old woman from a region with high prevalence of tuberculosis (South Asia) presents with blurring of vision and mild pain in both eyes for 3 months. Examination shows *bilateral granulomatous anterior uveitis* with 2+ cells, mutton-fat KPs, and posterior synechiae. Vitreous cells (1+) are present and there are a few choroidal spots in the periphery of the fundus. She also has a chronic cough and had unexplained fevers months ago. This presentation raises suspicion for *ocular tuberculosis* or sarcoidosis. Workup reveals a strongly positive IGRA test and a chest CT with apical fibrotic lesions consistent with prior TB infection. ACE level is mildly elevated. No organisms are found on sputum microscopy, but given the clinical picture, a diagnosis of presumed *tuberculous uveitis* is made (sarcoidosis is also possible, but in this epidemiologic context TB is more likely). The patient is started on a four-drug antituberculous therapy (ATT). After 2 weeks on ATT, oral prednisone 40 mg daily is added to suppress inflammation (started after initial antimicrobial cover) [22]. Over 2 months, her eyes quiet down to 0.5+ cells. The prednisone is tapered over 6 months, while ATT is continued for a total of 9 months. By treatment completion, she has 20/20 vision OU (both eyes) with no active inflammation. *Follow-up:* She was seen biweekly initially to monitor for paradoxical inflammatory worsening (which can happen in TB when starting therapy). Liver function tests were checked monthly due to ATT. Once stable, monthly eye examinations ensured no reactivation. This case underscores the importance of considering regional diseases in uveitis—the *epidemiologic context* (TB-endemic area) and *granulomatous signs* led to targeted TB testing, diagnosis, and appropriate therapy, resulting in cure of the uveitis.

Case 3—Masquerade syndrome (intraocular lymphoma): A 63-year-old woman with no significant medical history presents with gradual, painless blurring of vision in both eyes over 6 months. She was previously told she had "uveitis" and was given corticosteroid eye drops, which did not help. On examination, her best-corrected vision is 20/60 in each eye. Slit-lamp examination is unremarkable (no active anterior inflammation, but mild vitreous cells are noted on fundoscopy). Fundus examination shows a few creamy subretinal infiltrates in the periphery and mild vitritis. There is an impression of chorioretinal scarring. The uveitis appears *posterior, bilateral, and chronic*, but atypical in that it is relatively quiet in the anterior segment and *refractory to steroids*. Given her age, the differential includes a masquerade syndrome, such as primary vitreoretinal lymphoma (PVRL). An extensive infectious and autoimmune workup is unrevealing (syphilis, TB, sarcoid tests all negative; no systemic symptoms). Because of high suspicion, a diagnostic vitrectomy is performed. Cytology of the vitreous sample reveals large atypical lymphoid cells consistent with B-cell lymphoma, and molecular analysis finds an immunoglobulin H (IgH) gene rearrangement confirming clonality. She is diagnosed with *primary intraocular lymphoma* (a form of CNS lymphoma). The patient is started on systemic high-dose methotrexate chemotherapy combined with intravitreal methotrexate injections, in consultation with oncology. Remarkably, her ocular lesions resolve and vision improves to 20/30 in each eye. Unfortunately, 1 year later she develops CNS involvement (brain lesions), but enters remission after additional systemic chemotherapy. *Follow-up:* In the ophthalmic clinic, her inflammation was monitored monthly during active treatment, mainly by looking for recurrence of vitreous cells or new retinal lesions. This case highlights a masquerade syndrome—the keys were *older age, bilateral posterior uveitis unresponsive to intensive steroid therapy*, and test results excluding infection or autoimmune causes. The definitive diagnosis required an invasive test (vitreous biopsy) [30]. Management of such cases deviates from standard uveitis therapy and involves oncologic treatments.

Case 4—Infectious posterior uveitis (ocular toxoplasmosis): A 34-year-old woman presents with a 1-week history of blurred vision and floaters in her left eye. She describes seeing "cloudy spider webs" in that eye. She is otherwise healthy, with no systemic complaints. Visual acuity is 20/20 OD (right eye) and 20/50 OS (left eye). Anterior segments are normal, except for a few cells in the left anterior chamber. In the left vitreous, 2+ cells are noted (vitritis). Fundus examination of the left eye reveals a whitish-yellow retinal lesion with overlying haze located in the superotemporal quadrant, about one disc diameter in size, adjacent to a pigmented chorioretinal scar. There is mild optic disc edema. The right eye fundus is normal. This appearance is highly suggestive of *ocular toxoplasmosis*, where an old scar is reactivating with a new retinochoroiditis adjacent to it, accompanied by vitritis ("headlight in the fog" appearance). Infectious serologies confirmed high IgG titers for *Toxoplasma gondii* (IgM was negative, consistent with reactivation). No other infectious cause was found (syphilis non-reactive, negative IGRA). The patient was started on classic therapy for toxoplasmosis: oral pyrimethamine and sulfadiazine combined with folinic acid, along with prednisone 40 mg daily (started 48 hours after antimicrobials to avoid exacerbating the infection). After 6 weeks of therapy, the lesion healed into a scar and inflammation quieted. Her vision improved to 20/25 OS (left eye). Over the next 5 years, she had two additional reactivations at the border of the scar, each managed successfully with antimicrobial therapy (one time trimethoprim-sulfamethoxazole was used as an alternative regimen). She was subsequently placed on prophylactic trimethoprim-sulfamethoxazole (single strength daily) and has had no relapses in 3 years. *Discussion:* This case illustrates a common infectious uveitis. The hallmark of toxoplasmic uveitis is focal retinochoroiditis with dense vitritis (sometimes disproportionate to lesion size). The presence of an old scar strongly supports the diagnosis. Treatment requires specific antimicrobials to kill the parasite, with steroids used adjunctively to limit inflammation once therapy has begun. The case highlights the need to identify infection vs. autoimmunity; treating this with only steroids would have worsened the infection. Lifelong relapse potential in ocular toxoplasmosis means patients need counseling on recognizing symptoms early. Prophylactic therapy can be considered in cases with multiple relapses [1]. The prognosis in toxoplasmosis is good if the lesion is peripheral and managed promptly; however, lesions involving the macula or optic nerve carry a worse visual outcome. In this patient, the lesion was away from the macula and with appropriate therapy she sustained only minor visual loss. It demonstrates the principle that *identifying and treating the underlying cause* (here, a parasite) is crucial in uveitis care, and that long-term monitoring is necessary for recurrent conditions.

10. Recent advances and future directions

The field of uveitis has seen significant advances in both diagnostics and therapeutics, and ongoing research holds promise for improved patient outcomes:

- *Biologic therapies and targeted immunotherapy:* As discussed, TNF-α inhibitors like adalimumab have become game-changers for severe non-infectious uveitis, achieving remission in cases previously leading to blindness. Ongoing trials are exploring other pathways, such as IL-6 (with tocilizumab) and interleukin 17 (IL-17) (with secukinumab), and newer agents like janus kinase (JAK) inhibitors. Personalized medicine, where specific immune biomarkers could guide the choice of biologic, is an area of active investigation. Additionally, biosimilars (e.g., adalimumab biosimilars) are becoming available, expanding access to these therapies.

- *Intraocular sustained-release devices:* Corticosteroid implants (Retisert, Yutiq, Ozurdex) allow local long-term drug delivery. Upcoming technologies include biodegradable implants and refillable port delivery systems that might release immunomodulatory drugs, not just steroids. These can provide consistent therapy with fewer systemic effects. Research is also looking at drug-eluting suprachoroidal implants for even more targeted therapy.

- *Gene therapy:* Uveitis is being explored as a candidate for gene therapy to induce local production of anti-inflammatory molecules. Preclinical studies have tried viral vectors that deliver genes for IL-10 or soluble TNF receptors to the eye. The idea is a one-time treatment could confer long-term protection against uveitis flares by locally altering the immune response. Challenges include ensuring safety of vectors and avoiding unwanted inflammation from the gene delivery itself. While not yet in clinical use for uveitis, gene therapy remains a future avenue for refractory cases [31].

- *Novel imaging and diagnostics:* Advanced imaging like OCT angiography (OCTA) (which can detect retinal vascular changes without dye) and ultra-widefield fluorescein angiography (UWFA) are enhancing our ability to see peripheral retinal vasculitis and quantify non-perfusion. These technologies will likely become routine in uveitis clinics. Additionally, proteomic and metabolomic analyses of aqueous humor are being studied to identify unique "fingerprints" of certain uveitic entities, which could 1 day allow a rapid laboratory test to diagnose, say, sarcoid uveitis by analyzing a small fluid sample. A multiplex PCR panel on intraocular fluid (for infectious uveitis pathogens) is an emerging diagnostic that could simultaneously test for herpes viruses, *Toxoplasma*, and *Mycobacterium* in one go, aiding prompt etiological diagnosis.

- *Clinical guidelines and care models:* There is a push toward standardized care pathways, such as the aforementioned international *FOCUS* guidelines [23] for immunosuppression in uveitis and consensus guidelines for specific diseases (e.g., the *SUN Working Group* has published classification criteria for uveitides to standardize research and practice) [8]. These efforts improve consistency of care. Multicenter studies (like the Multicenter Uveitis Steroid Treatment (MUST) trial for systemic vs. implant therapy in uveitis) inform best practices. The trend is toward earlier introduction of IMT, tight control of inflammation (treat-to-target of zero cells), and careful monitoring, analogous to approaches in rheumatoid arthritis.

- *Future challenges:* Despite advances, management of uveitis in resource-limited settings remains challenging, as does uveitis in pediatric patients who may have lifelong disease. Also, certain diseases like serpiginous choroiditis or multifocal choroiditis still lack highly effective targeted therapies. Ongoing research into the pathogenesis of uveitis (including the microbiome's role in HLA-B27 disease or genetic predispositions) may unveil new treatment targets. The integration of *telemedicine* for monitoring quiescent patients with remote OCTs or apps to assess vision is also a potential future direction, to catch relapses early.

In conclusion, the outlook for uveitis patients has never been better. With a combination of modern immunotherapy, cutting-edge imaging, and a systematic clinical approach, we can preserve vision in the vast majority of uveitis cases. The coming years promise further refinements, including possibly remission-inducing treatments (or even cures) through gene therapy or highly specific immune modulation. Multidisciplinary care and patient education will remain cornerstones, ensuring that these advances translate into real-world success. Subsequent chapters will explore the role of anterior segment optical coherence tomography in uveitis [15], clinical features and management of Vogt-Koyanagi-Harada disease [11], Behçet's disease [6], ocular tuberculosis, use of glaucoma drainage implants in uveitic glaucoma [24], and the specific challenges of managing uveitis in low- to middle-income countries.

11. Conclusion

Uveitis encompasses a broad range of intraocular inflammatory diseases that require prompt recognition and a careful, systematic approach to management. By classifying uveitis accurately and investigating pertinent causes, clinicians can tailor therapy to the individual patient. The cornerstone of treatment is controlling inflammation, primarily with corticosteroids and supplemented by immunomodulatory therapy in chronic or severe cases to achieve steroid-sparing remission. Equally important is the management of any underlying systemic disease or infection in tandem with ocular therapy. Advances in imaging (OCT, FFA, AS-OCT) have enhanced our ability to monitor disease activity and guide treatment decisions. Through illustrative cases, we see how an evidence-based approach—from diagnosis through follow-up—can lead to successful outcomes, even in potentially blinding uveitis. Interdisciplinary collaboration (with rheumatology, infectious disease, etc.) often improves diagnostic accuracy and patient care, reflecting the systemic nature uveitis can have.

While challenges remain, the progress in uveitis management over recent years has greatly improved prognosis for patients. Vision loss from uveitis is no longer inevitable in many cases, as long as appropriate therapy is instituted and maintained. The key is to *individualize treatment*: some patients may do well with topical steroids alone, whereas others require aggressive multi-agent systemic therapy; some cases resolve after a finite course, while others need long-term maintenance. Physicians must remain vigilant in follow-up to detect relapses or complications early and adjust treatment accordingly.

In summary, the management of uveitis is complex but rewarding—by quelling ocular inflammation and addressing its root causes, we preserve sight and improve quality of life. This chapter has provided a comprehensive overview of diagnostic and therapeutic strategies in uveitis. Building on this foundation, the following chapters will explore specific imaging modalities and advanced therapies that continue to evolve, further equipping clinicians to tackle uveitis with confidence and expertise.

Acknowledgements

This chapter benefited from language refinement using ChatGPT (OpenAI, San Francisco, CA, USA), under the direction of the author.

Conflict of interest

The authors declare no conflict of interest.

Author details

Seema Rani[1] and Joobin Khadamy[2]*

1 Department of Ophthalmology, Government Medical College (GMC), Udhampur, India

2 Department of Ophthalmology, University Hospital of Umea, Umea, Sweden

*Address all correspondence to: joobin.khadamy@regionvasterbotten.se

References

[1] Tuğal-Tutkun İ. An overview of pediatric uveitis. Turkish Archives of Pediatrics. 2023;**58**:363-370

[2] Gritz DC, Wong IG. Incidence and prevalence of uveitis in northern California; the northern California epidemiology of uveitis study. Ophthalmology. 2004;**111**:491-500 discussion 500

[3] Akinsoji E, Goldhardt R, Galor A. A glimpse into uveitis in the aging eye: Pathophysiology, clinical presentation and treatment considerations. Drugs & Aging. 2018;**35**:399-408

[4] Rathinam SR, Namperumalsamy P. Global variation and pattern changes in epidemiology of uveitis. Indian Journal of Ophthalmology. 2007;**55**:173-183

[5] González MM, Solano MM, Porco TC, et al. Epidemiology of uveitis in a US population-based study. Journal of Ophthalmic Inflammation and Infection. 2018;**8**:6

[6] Köksaldı S. Ocular Involvement in Behçet's Disease. London, UK: IntechOpen; 2025

[7] Gul Malik T, Ul Ain N. Perspective chapter: Challenges in managing uveitis in low- to middle-income countries. In: Khadamy MDJ, editor. Uveitis in the Clinic – Current Approaches and Future Directions in Diagnosis, Treatment, and Patient Care. London, UK: IntechOpen; 2025

[8] Jabs DA, Nussenblatt RB, Rosenbaum JT, et al. Standardization of uveitis nomenclature for reporting clinical data. Results of the first international workshop. American Journal of Ophthalmology. 2005;**140**:509-516

[9] Nussenblatt RB, Palestine AG, Chan CC, et al. Standardization of vitreal inflammatory activity in intermediate and posterior uveitis. Ophthalmology. 1985;**92**:467-471

[10] Arepalli S. Current Diagnosis and Management of Uveitis. Review of Ophthalmology. Thorofare, NJ, USA: Jobson Medical Information LLC; 14 Sep 2022. Available from: https://www.reviewofophthalmology.com/article/current-diagnosis-and-management-of-uveitis [Accessed: April 27, 2025]

[11] Kayabaşı M. Clinical features and treatment options of Vogt-Koyanagi-Harada disease. In: Khadamy MDJ, editor. Uveitis in the Clinic – Current Approaches and Future Directions in Diagnosis, Treatment, and Patient Care. London, UK: IntechOpen; 2025

[12] Onal S, Tugal-Tutkun I, Neri P, et al. Optical coherence tomography imaging in uveitis. International Ophthalmology. 2014;**34**:401-435

[13] Gupta V, Al-Dhibi HA, Arevalo JF. Retinal imaging in uveitis. Saudi Journal of Ophthalmology. 2014;**28**(2):95-103. DOI: 10.1016/j.sjopt.2014.02.008

[14] Khadamy J. Anterior-segment optical coherence tomography unlocks novel perspectives: Lacking iris anterior limiting layer signal in uveitis. Cureus. 2024;**16**:e51872

[15] Khadamy J. Anterior segment optical coherence tomography in uveitis: Current applications and future directions. In: Khadamy MDJ, editor. Uveitis in the Clinic – Current Approaches and Future Directions in Diagnosis, Treatment, and Patient Care. London, UK: IntechOpen; 2025

[16] Ness T, Boehringer D, Heinzelmann S. Intermediate uveitis: Pattern of etiology, complications, treatment and outcome in a tertiary academic center. Orphanet Journal of Rare Diseases. 2017;**12**:81

[17] Treatment of Uveitis – EyeWiki. 2023. Available from: https://eyewiki.org/Treatment_of_Uveitis#:~:text=Inferior%20Transseptal%20Approach [Accessed: April 27, 2025]

[18] Jabs DA. Immunosuppression for the uveitides. Ophthalmology. 2018;**125**:193-202

[19] Dahr SS. A Long-Term Game Plan for Noninfectious Uveitis. Retina Specialist. Thorofare, NJ, USA: Jobson Medical Information LLC; 29 Jun 2017. Available from: https://www.retina-specialist.com/article/a-longterm-game-plan-for-noninfectious-uveitis [Accessed: April 27, 2025]

[20] Valdes LM, Sobrin L. Uveitis therapy: The corticosteroid options. Drugs. 2020;**80**:765-773

[21] Tirelli F, Zannin ME, Vittadello F, et al. Methotrexate monotherapy in juvenile idiopathic arthritis associated uveitis: Myth or reality? Ocular Immunology and Inflammation. 2022;**30**:1763-1767

[22] Agrawal H, Doan H, Pham B, et al. Systemic immunosuppressive therapies for uveitis in developing countries. Indian Journal of Ophthalmology. 2020;**68**:1852-1862

[23] Dick AD, Rosenbaum JT, Al-Dhibi HA, et al. Guidance on noncorticosteroid systemic immunomodulatory therapy in noninfectious uveitis: Fundamentals of care for UveitiS (FOCUS) initiative. Ophthalmology. 2018;**125**:757-773

[24] Besozzi G, Santoro M, Cassano F, et al. Glaucoma drainage implants for uveitic glaucoma. In: Khadamy MDJ, editor. Uveitis in the Clinic – Current Approaches and Future Directions in Diagnosis, Treatment, and Patient Care. London, UK: IntechOpen; 2025

[25] Cunningham ET, Yamamoto JH, Arevalo JF, et al. Retinal detachment in uveitis. Ocular Immunology and Inflammation. 2023;**31**:1-2

[26] Clowse ME, Förger F, Hwang C, et al. Minimal to no transfer of certolizumab pegol into breast milk: Results from CRADLE, a prospective, postmarketing, multicentre, pharmacokinetic study. Annals of the Rheumatic Diseases. 2017;**76**:1890-1896

[27] Chiam NPY, Lim LLP. Uveitis and gender: The course of uveitis in pregnancy. Journal of Ophthalmology. 2014;**2014**:401915

[28] Maccora I, Simonini G, Guly CM, et al. Management of JIA associated uveitis. Best Practice & Research. Clinical Rheumatology. 2024;**38**:101979

[29] David Holland OD. Ordering and Interpretation of Uveitis Work-Up. San Diego, CA, USA: Eyes On Eyecare; 2023. Available from: https://eyesoneyecare.com/resources/ordering-and-interpretation-of-uveitis-work-up/ [Accessed: April 27, 2025]

[30] Harman LE, Margo CE, Roetzheim RG. Uveitis: The collaborative diagnostic evaluation. American Family Physician. 2014;**90**:711-716

[31] Liu MM, Tuo J, Chan C-C. Gene therapy for ocular diseases. The British Journal of Ophthalmology. 2011;**95**:604-612

Chapter 2

Anterior Segment Optical Coherence Tomography in Uveitis: Current Applications and Future Directions

Joobin Khadamy

Abstract

Anterior segment optical coherence tomography (AS-OCT) is a non-invasive imaging modality providing high-resolution images of anterior ocular structures, aiding morphological assessments and biomarker identification in uveitis management. This chapter examines AS-OCT's clinical and investigational roles in uveitis, detailing its utility in detecting subtle corneal changes, keratic precipitate (KP) morphology, anterior chamber cells, and iris structural alterations. AS-OCT facilitates longitudinal monitoring of anterior uveal inflammation, mirroring histopathological changes *in vivo*. It distinguishes granulomatous from non-granulomatous KPs, supports evaluation of infectious uveitis subtypes, and assesses angle structures for trabeculitis or synechiae-related glaucoma. Pre- and post-cataract surgery assessments in complex uveitic cases benefit significantly from AS-OCT, aiding differentiation of conditions such as Posner-Schlossman syndrome and Fuchs' uveitis syndrome *via* iris morphology analysis. Despite its advantages, AS-OCT faces technical limitations, including suboptimal visualization of iris, posterior chamber, ciliary body, and middle segment—though this can be partially addressed using contact lens-assisted imaging—difficulty differentiating inflammatory cells from pigment or debris, and susceptibility to artifacts. Emerging innovations like spectroscopic OCT (SOCT) for molecular profiling, pseudocolor segmentation, adaptive optics OCT (AO-OCT), and robotic-assisted imaging promise artifact-free acquisition and enhanced resolution. Integration with complementary technologies like laser flare photometry (LFP), ultrasound biomicroscopy (UBM), confocal microscopy, and radiomics-based AI analytics strengthens multimodal imaging approaches. Advancing these combined modalities promotes standardized diagnostics, biomarker development—including molecular, cellular, and structural biomarkers—and fully automated, precision-driven uveitis care.

Keywords: anterior segment optical coherence tomography (AS-OCT), uveitis management, non-invasive imaging, morphological assessment, biomarker identification, keratic precipitate morphology, anterior chamber inflammation, middle segment imaging, spectroscopic OCT, adaptive optics

1. Introduction

Uveitis is a complex, vision-threatening inflammatory condition characterized by diverse etiologies and variable clinical presentations. Traditional methods, such as slit-lamp examination (SLE) and gonioscopy, are limited by subjectivity and impaired visualization in media opacities. AS-OCT helps overcome these challenges by providing high-resolution, cross-sectional imaging of the anterior segment (including the cornea, anterior chamber (AC), iris, and lens), enabling objective, quantitative assessment [1, 2].

Advances in swept-source OCT, offering axial resolutions of 3–5 μm, combined with AI-driven analytics, have enabled the detection of subtle histopathophysiological changes [3]. However, imaging of the ciliary body (CB) and posterior chamber (PC) remains suboptimal, and differentiating pigment from inflammatory cells is still problematic. This chapter details these advances and limitations while discussing the emerging need for middle-segment imaging and color-coded OCT [4]—essential for the next generation of uveitis diagnostics in the era of AI and robotics [5, 6].

This chapter is a narrative review combining literature evidence with clinical AS-OCT cases obtained using the Topcon Triton Swept-Source AS-OCT. A literature search was performed on PubMed using the terms: ("AS-OCT" OR "Anterior Segment Optical Coherence Tomography" OR "Anterior Segment Imaging") AND ("Uveitis" OR "Iritis" OR "Ocular Inflammation"), supplemented by manual reference checking to identify relevant publications. Written or oral informed consent was obtained from all patients whose clinical or imaging data were included. Histopathological samples were not obtained, as non-invasive imaging provided sufficient diagnostic information in all cases. Clinical slit-lamp photographs were included when available to correlate with AS-OCT images; however, infrared (IR) reference images were excluded due to their limited resolution and minimal interpretive value.

2. Technical principles of AS-OCT and innovations

2.1 AS-OCT fundamentals

AS-OCT employs low-coherence interferometry with near-infrared light (typically around 1310 nm) to produce high-resolution cross-sectional images. Modern swept-source systems, capable of up to 100,000 A-scans per second, reduce motion artifacts—a key advantage in uncooperative or pediatric patients. However, most devices are optimized for the cornea and AC, limiting their performance in imaging the CB and PC [7, 8].

2.2 Spectroscopic and color-coded OCT

Spectroscopic OCT (SOCT) and true/pseudocolor-coded OCT represent emerging advancements in optical coherence tomography that enhance the diagnostic capabilities of conventional OCT systems. Spectroscopic OCT analyzes the wavelength-dependent scattering properties of tissues, providing molecular and biochemical insights that can differentiate inflammatory cells, pigment granules, and exudates—key challenges in uveitis imaging. This technique holds promise for identifying specific biomarkers, such as protein composition in keratic precipitates (KPs) or distinguishing granulomatous from non-granulomatous inflammation. True/color-coded OCT, on the other hand, assigns different colors to various tissue layers and structures based on their reflectivity or scattering profiles, improving visualization and interpretation of complex anatomical features like iris nodules, synechiae, or angle abnormalities [4]. True color OCT refers to imaging techniques that capture actual spectral color data, as opposed to pseudocolor reflectivity mapping. By enhancing contrast and providing intuitive visual cues, color-coded OCT facilitates the detection of subtle changes in the anterior segment, iris (**Figures 1** and **2**), and posterior uveitis. Together, these technologies have the potential to overcome the limitations of

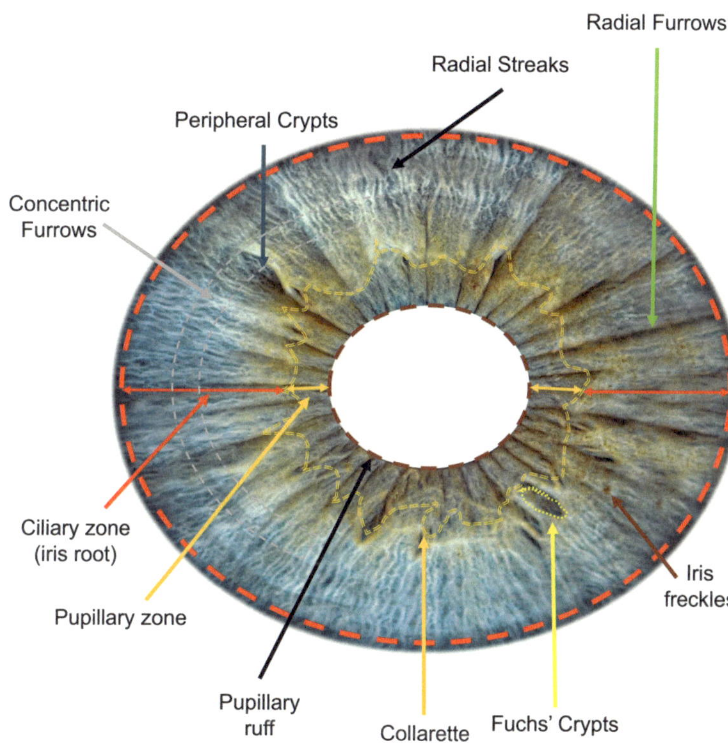

Figure 1.
Anatomical features of the human iris, highlighting key structural zones and landmarks. The pupillary zone (inner region) and ciliary zone (outer region) are separated by the collarette, the thickest part of the iris, which marks the boundary between the pupillary and ciliary portions. The pupillary ruff surrounds the pupil with a dark, pigmented edge. Fuchs' crypts, visible as irregular openings near the collarette, allow aqueous humor to be exchanged within the iris stroma. The peripheral crypts are located near the iris root at the outermost edge. Radial furrows and radial streaks run outward from the pupil, forming structural support for iris dilation and contraction. Concentric furrows are visible in the ciliary zone, aiding in iris folding during pupillary movement. Iris freckles, small pigmented spots, can be seen scattered across the surface. These anatomical features play essential roles in iris function and clinical evaluation in ocular conditions such as uveitis, glaucoma, iris cysts, or uveal tumors.

grayscale imaging, offering more precise diagnostics and paving the way for personalized uveitis management. It is noteworthy that spectroscopic and true/color-coded OCT technologies are currently in the research phase and are not yet widely available for clinical use.

2.3 AI and robotic integration in AS-OCT

The integration of artificial intelligence (AI) and robotic technology with anterior segment optical coherence tomography (AS-OCT) is revolutionizing ocular imaging by enhancing precision, automation, and accessibility. AI algorithms enable automated segmentation of anterior segment structures, such as the cornea, iris, and angle, improving the accuracy of inflammation quantification (e.g., anterior chamber cell and flare grading) while reducing interobserver variability. One of AI's most transformative roles in AS-OCT is artifact correction. Common artifacts such as motion blur, shadowing from dense KPs, mirror artifacts from corneal reflections,

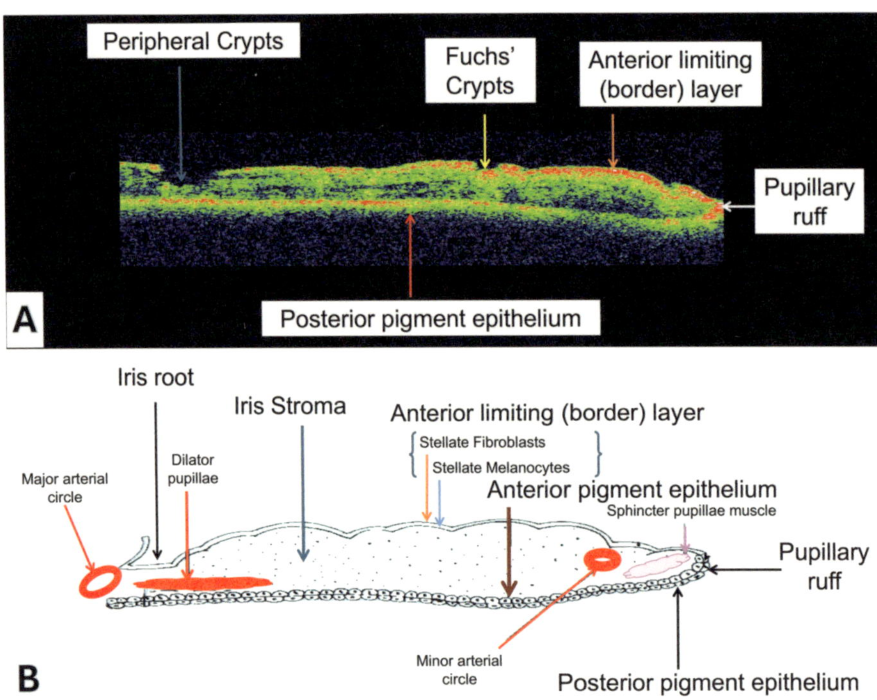

Figure 2.
High-resolution AS-OCT imaging and schematic representation of the iris anatomy. (A) Anterior segment optical coherence tomography (AS-OCT) image of the human iris, highlighting key structural features. The peripheral crypts, located near the iris root, facilitate aqueous humor exchange, while Fuchs' crypts, irregular openings near the collarette, aid in fluid dynamics within the iris stroma. The anterior limiting (border) layer, composed of stellate fibroblasts and melanocytes, provides structural support and pigmentation. The highly reflective posterior pigment epithelium absorbs light and prevents stray light scattering, contributing to visual clarity. The pupillary ruff, a pigmented edge around the pupil, is formed by the posterior pigment epithelium folding forward. (B) Schematic diagram of the iris anatomy, illustrating its layers and vascular structures. The iris root connects the iris to the ciliary body, while the iris stroma contains blood vessels, nerves, and connective tissue. The major arterial circle, located near the iris root, supplies blood to the stroma, branching into smaller vessels forming the minor arterial circle near the collarette. The sphincter pupillae muscle, situated near the pupillary margin, is responsible for pupillary constriction, while the dilator pupillae muscle facilitates dilation. Together, these images provide detailed insights into iris structure and function as visualized by AS-OCT and anatomical schematics.

and saturation artifacts caused by hyperreflective surfaces can obscure critical details in uveitis imaging. AI-driven algorithms can detect and suppress these artifacts by analyzing signal patterns, reconstructing missing data, and differentiating true anatomical structures from noise. For example, deep learning models trained on large datasets can distinguish inflammatory cells from pigment granules or debris, a key challenge in uveitis diagnosis [6]. Robotic assistance in AS-OCT typically refers to motorized alignment systems and real-time eye tracking. Robotic systems further enhance AS-OCT by automating scan alignment and real-time eye tracking [9], minimizing motion artifacts, and ensuring consistent image quality. These advancements streamline image acquisition workflows and expand access to high-quality imaging in underserved areas through telemedicine platforms. The integration of AI-based artifact correction and robotic precision positions AS-OCT as a candidate for fully automated diagnostics capable of delivering standardized, artifact-free imaging for precise automated uveitis management. It is important to note that many AI applications in ophthalmic imaging, including those involving AS-OCT, remain in the prototype or clinical validation phase and are not yet integrated into standard clinical care. Current limitations of AI algorithms in AS-OCT include the need for larger labeled datasets, regulatory and ethical considerations, and validation through extensive clinical trials.

2.4 Comparative analysis of imaging modalities

Uveitis evaluation requires diverse imaging modalities, each optimized for specific anatomical regions and clinical goals. From foundational tools like slit lamp examination (SLE) and laser flare photometry (LFP) to advanced technologies such as adaptive optics OCT (AO-OCT), swept-source OCT (SS-OCT) [10], and ultrasound (US), these modalities offer unique strengths and limitations. SLE remains the gold standard for initial clinical grading of AC inflammation, LFP objectively quantifies aqueous flare, it cannot distinguish cell morphology or location, an area where AS-OCT provides complementary value. AS-OCT has revolutionized anterior segment imaging with its high resolution [11], but its limited penetration depth necessitates complementary tools like ultrasound biomicroscopy (UBM) and US for deeper structures such as the CB and pars plana [12]. Swept-Source OCT uses a longer wavelength (~1050 nm) and tunable laser to achieve faster scan speeds and deeper tissue penetration, making it ideal for imaging the choroid and vitreous in posterior uveitis. Emerging technologies like AO-OCT offer experimental applications for cellular-level visualization of the iris and trabecular meshwork. AO-OCT employs real-time correction of optical aberrations to provide near-cellular-level resolution, enabling detailed visualization of microstructures [10]. For posterior uveitis, modalities such as fundus fluorescein angiography (FFA), indocyanine green angiography (ICGA), SS-OCT, and US remain indispensable for evaluating retinal, choroidal, and vitreous involvement [13]. Swept-source OCT (SS-OCT) systems use longer wavelengths (~1050 nm), allowing deeper tissue penetration, while Adaptive Optics OCT (AO-OCT) typically uses similar near-infrared light (~800–900 nm) but incorporates real-time correction for optical aberrations to achieve near-cellular resolution. **Table 1** provides a comprehensive comparison of these imaging modalities, highlighting their resolution, penetration depth, key applications, limitations, and clinical relevance in uveitis care. It highlights the gold standard tools for specific tasks (e.g., LFP for flare quantification and UBM for ciliary body imaging). AS-OCTA and AO-OCT represent emerging technologies that offer unprecedented detail at the microvascular and cellular levels.

Modality	Resolution	Penetration Depth	Key Structures Imaged	Applications & Limitations
SLE	Low (~10–20 μm)	Entire anterior segment	Inflammatory cells, keratic precipitates (KPs), angle (with gonioscopy)	Gold standard for clinical grading of anterior chamber inflammation; widely available and inexpensive but subjective grading with interobserver variability; lacks cellular-level detail.
LFP	Low (~100 μm for flare quantification)	Anterior chamber only	Quantifies aqueous flare intensity (protein concentration surrogate)	Gold standard for objective flare quantification in anterior uveitis; fast and reproducible, but cannot visualize inflammatory cells or structural changes.
AS-OCT	High (~5–10 μm)	Cornea to lens (~2–3 mm)	Inflammatory cells, KPs, synechiae, and angle structures	Invetigational for anterior chamber inflammation quantification; synechiae monitoring; KP analysis; widely available but moderately expensive; limited penetration depth; artifacts (motion blur and shadowing); no ciliary body visualization.
UBM	Moderate (~20–50 μm)	Good for Ciliary body (CB), pars plana (PP) (~5–10 mm)	CB, PP; effective through opaque media	Gold standard for CB and PP imaging; posterior chamber assessment; widely available but requires contact with the eye; lower resolution compared to AS-OCT.
IVCM	Very high (~1 μm lateral)	Cornea (~0.5–0.6 mm)	Cellular details of KPs, endothelial cells	Gold standard for cellular-level analysis of KPs and endothelial plaques; requires contact with the eye; less commonly available due to high cost; limited depth penetration and small field of view; slower acquisition speeds compared to AS-OCT.
AO-OCT	Very high (~1–3 μm)	Limited (~2 mm)	Iris crypts, melanocytes, trabecular meshwork	Experimental use in anterior segment research; not widely adopted clinically due to high cost and limited availability; offers cellular-level resolution but is not optimized for routine anterior segment imaging.
AS-OCTA	High (~5–10 μm)	Anterior segment	Blood vessels in iris/angle	Vascular imaging in iris neovascularization or vasculitis; limited adoption due to high cost and motion artifacts during acquisition.

Modality	Resolution	Penetration Depth	Key Structures Imaged	Applications & Limitations
SS-OCT	High (~5–10 μm axial resolution)	Posterior segment (~6–13 mm)	Retina, choroid, optic nerve head	Imaging retinal layers and choroidal structures in posterior uveitis; commonly available but not optimized for anterior segment imaging.
FFA	Moderate (~20 μm)	Posterior segment	Retinal/choroidal vessels	Gold standard for posterior uveitis; vasculitis, and choroiditis imaging; commonly available but requires intravenous dye injection with moderate resolution compared to OCT-based modalities.
ICGA	Moderate (~20 μm axial resolution)	Posterior segment to choroid (~300 μm depth penetration)	Choroidal vessels and deep retinal vasculature	Gold standard for imaging choroiditis and posterior uveitis with choroidal vascular involvement; commonly available but invasive due to intravenous dye injection with moderate resolution.
US	Moderate (~100–200 μm axial resolution)	Deep penetration (~10–15 mm)	Vitreous opacities, retinal detachment, posterior segment masses	Commonly used for detecting vitreous opacities, serous retinal detachment, and choroidal masses in posterior uveitis; effective through opaque media but lower resolution than OCT-based modalities.

SLE: Slit Lamp Examination; LFP: Laser Flare Photometry; AS-OCT: Anterior Segment Optical Coherence Tomography; UBM: Ultrasound Biomicroscopy; IVCM: In Vivo Confocal Microscopy; AO-OCT: Adaptive Optics Optical Coherence Tomography; AS-OCTA: Anterior Segment OCT Angiography; FFA: Fundus Fluorescein Angiography; ICGA: Indocyanine Green Angiography; US: Ultrasound (B-scan); SS-OCT: Swept-Source Optical Coherence Tomography; KP: Keratic Precipitates.

Table 1.
Comparative analysis of imaging modalities for uveitis evaluation.

2.5 Comparative analysis of commercial AS-OCT and AS-OCTA devices in uveitis

Commercial AS-OCT and anterior segment OCT angiography (AS-OCTA) devices offer a wide range of capabilities for imaging the anterior segment (**Table 2**), each catering to specific clinical needs in uveitis management. While AS-OCT and AS-OCTA devices offer significant advantages in imaging the anterior segment, understanding their specific features and limitations is crucial for optimal use in clinical practice.

AS-OCT devices, such as the CASIA2 (Tomey Corporation, Nagoya, Japan) and Spectralis (Heidelberg Engineering, Heidelberg, Germany), are primarily designed for corneal topography and tomography, excelling in high-resolution imaging of the cornea, AC, and angle structures. The CASIA2, with its wide scan diameter of up to 16 mm and a scanning depth of 13 mm, is particularly well-suited for angle imaging due to its automated angle analysis and comprehensive field of view. In contrast, the

Device	Type and technology	Resolution and scan diameter	Key features	Strengths	Limitations
CASIA2 (Tomey)	AS-OCT (SS- OCT)	10 µm axial, ~20 µm lateral, Up to 16 mm (scan depth to 13 mm)	Wide-angle scanning; automated angle analysis; corneal topography and tomography	Excellent for angle imaging; wide field of view; ideal for corneal and anterior chamber analysis	Not optimized for iris imaging; lacks pseudocolor or true color-coded imaging capabilities
Spectralis (Heidelberg)	AS-OCT (SD-OCT)	3.9 µm axial, 5.7 µm lateral, 6 mm	Enhanced resolution for structural imaging; multimodal capabilities with posterior segment OCT	Superior structural detail for iris imaging; integrates with posterior segment imaging systems	Limited penetration depth (~2–3 mm); cannot visualize deeper structures like the ciliary body
Optovue Avanti	AS-OCT/ AS-OCTA (SD-OCT, High-Speed)	5 µm axial, ~10 µm lateral, 6 mm	Combines AS-OCT and AS-OCTA; pseudocolor-coded maps for corneal epithelial thickness	Versatile device for both structural and vascular imaging; pseudocolor-coded maps enhance corneal diagnostics	Prone to motion artifacts in AS-OCTA mode; higher cost compared to standalone AS-OCT devices
Triton DRI OCT (Topcon)	SS-OCTA (SS-OCT)	8 µm axial, ~20 µm lateral, 6 mm	Swept-Source technology; color-coded vascular maps; deep penetration (~6–13 mm)	Advanced vascular imaging for detecting iris neovascularization or vasculitis; color-coded vascular maps	Primarily designed for posterior segment imaging; limited optimization for anterior segment structures
MS-39 (CSO)	AS-OCT (SD-OCT)	10 µm axial, ~20 µm lateral, 9–10 mm	Corneal tomography and anterior chamber depth mapping with pseudocolor-coded maps	Excellent for corneal diagnostics; pseudocolor-coded maps improve visualization of thickness and depth parameters	Lacks vascular imaging capabilities; not optimized for iris-specific studies
Cirrus HD-OCT 5000 (Zeiss)	AS-OCT (SD-OCT)	5 µm axial, ~10 µm lateral, 6 mm	High-resolution anterior segment and posterior segment imaging	Reliable for corneal and anterior chamber analysis; integrates with posterior OCT systems	Limited field of view for wide-angle imaging; lacks vascular imaging capabilities

Device	Type and technology	Resolution and scan diameter	Key features	Strengths	Limitations
PLEX Elite 9000 (Zeiss)	SS-OCTA (SS-OCT)	6.3 μm axial, ~20 μm lateral, Up to 12 mm	Swept-Source OCT Angiography with deep penetration and wide-field scanning	Excellent for vascular imaging in the iris, angle, and posterior segment; large scan diameter	High cost; primarily designed for research settings rather than routine clinical use
ANTERION (Heidelberg)	AS-OCT (SS-OCT)	~10 μm axial, ~20 μm lateral, Up to 16.5 mm	Combines biometry, corneal topography, tomography, and anterior chamber analysis	Wide scan diameter ideal for comprehensive anterior segment evaluation, including angle and lens imaging	High cost; not optimized for vascular imaging or detailed iris analysis

AS-OCT: Anterior Segment Optical Coherence Tomography; SS-OCTA: Swept-Source Optical Coherence Tomography Angiography; AS-OCTA: Anterior Segment Optical Coherence Tomography Angiography; SD-OCT: Spectral-Domain Optical Coherence Tomography.

Table 2.
Comparative analysis of commercial AS-OCT and AS-OCTA devices in uveitis.

Spectralis provides enhanced resolution (~4 μm axial) that is better suited for detailed structural imaging of the iris. The Spectralis is primarily used for retinal imaging but has capabilities for anterior segment imaging. It features TruTrack active eye tracking, which minimizes motion artifacts. Devices like the MS-39 (CSO, Florence, Italy) and ANTERION (Heidelberg Engineering, Heidelberg, Germany) also focus on corneal diagnostics, offering pseudocolor-coded maps for epithelial thickness and anterior chamber depth (ACD), which can be useful in uveitis cases involving secondary corneal changes.

AS-OCTA devices, such as the Optovue Avanti (Optovue Inc., Fremont, CA, USA), Triton DRI OCT (Topcon Corporation, Tokyo, Japan), and PLEX Elite 9000 (Carl Zeiss Meditec, Dublin, CA, USA), add a functional dimension by visualizing blood flow in the iris and angle. Optovue Avanti is a spectral-domain OCT system with wide-field capabilities that is suitable for both posterior and anterior segment imaging. It offers a scan area of up to 12 mm x 9 mm. These systems are particularly valuable for detecting vascular abnormalities such as iris neovascularization or vasculitis in uveitis cases with suspected vascular involvement. It offers high-speed scanning and deep penetration. The PLEX Elite 9000 stands out with its large scan diameter of up to 12 mm, making it ideal for wide-field vascular imaging. This device is primarily focused on posterior segment imaging, but can be used for AS-OCTA with appropriate adaptors. Similarly, the Triton DRI OCT offers color-coded vascular maps alongside deep penetration (~6–13 mm), enabling visualization of blood flow abnormalities in both anterior and posterior segments. However, AS-OCTA devices are more prone to motion artifacts during vascular imaging and have limited adoption due to higher costs and a lack of standardized protocols, though validation studies are currently in progress.

A significant limitation of many AS-OCT systems lies in their scan pattern configuration, where Y-plane reconstructions or volumetric images are derived from sequential X-plane B-scans rather than being directly acquired. While this method is standard in OCT imaging, misalignment during acquisition can contribute to artifacts—most notably mirror artifacts, particularly in Fourier-domain OCT systems, in which highly reflective structures such as the cornea or iris may appear inverted or duplicated within the AC, potentially obscuring critical anatomical landmarks like the iris contour or angle structures [14]. Furthermore, most commercially available AS-OCT devices are optimized for corneal and AC assessment, with scan diameter, axial resolution, and focal depth primarily configured for these regions. As a result, they are not specifically designed for high-resolution iris imaging, which limits the ability to evaluate iris-based pathology in detail. Devices like the CASIA2 and ANTERION address this limitation by offering larger scan diameters (up to 16–16.5 mm), which improve wide-angle imaging of anterior segment structures.

For corneal-focused applications like topography or tomography, devices such as the CASIA2, MS-39, and ANTERION remain the gold standard due to their wide field of view and pseudocolor-coded mapping capabilities. For detailed structural analysis of the iris or angle in inflammatory conditions, systems like Spectralis or CASIA2 are preferred due to their high resolution. On the other hand, for vascular assessments in cases of ischemia or neovascular complications, AS-OCTA devices like Optovue Avanti or PLEX Elite 9000 offer en face vascular imaging of the iris and limbal region, enabling visualization of neovascularization and vessel remodeling in anterior segment inflammation. While still investigational in uveitis, these systems hold potential for non-invasive vascular biomarker assessment. Future advancements should focus on optimizing scan patterns for iris-specific imaging, minimizing artifacts such as mirror reflections, and integrating advanced pseudocolor visualization tools to enhance diagnostic accuracy in uveitis care.

Table 2 presents a comparison of commercial AS-OCT and AS-OCTA devices, highlighting their technological features, resolutions, key capabilities, strengths, and limitations. Overall, each device caters to specific clinical needs in uveitis management, emphasizing the importance of selecting the appropriate device based on diagnostic requirements. The values provided in the table are based on available data from manufacturer specifications and relevant literature. While efforts have been made to ensure accuracy, some values, particularly lateral resolutions, may not be explicitly stated in all sources. For devices like the Spectralis, detailed studies have confirmed lateral resolutions around 5.7 μm, while other devices may have estimates based on typical OCT technology. Axial resolution determines the ability to distinguish between structures at different depths, while lateral resolution affects the ability to differentiate between structures side by side. Higher resolutions in both dimensions enhance diagnostic accuracy by providing more detailed images.

3. Clinical applications of AS-OCT in uveitis

Anterior AS-OCT has transformed the diagnosis and management of uveitis by providing high-resolution, non-invasive imaging of the anterior segment. This technology not only enhances our ability to detect subtle structural changes but also bridges the gap between clinical observation and underlying histopathological processes. In the following sections, we detail the various clinical applications of AS-OCT in uveitis, covering histopathological insights, corneal assessments, AC inflammation, iris, and pupillary changes, angle evaluation for glaucoma mechanisms, lens and cataract evaluation, and anterior vitreous inflammation. Useful tables summarizing key findings and clinical implications are provided at the end.

3.1 *In vivo* clinical histopathological insights in uveitis

Anterior AS-OCT offers an unprecedented *in vivo* window into the histopathological events in uveitis. By capturing longitudinal dynamic changes that bridge traditional static histology and evolving clinical conditions, AS-OCT provides detailed insights into cellular and structural alterations—shedding light on the mechanisms of inflammation, adhesion formation, and tissue remodeling (**Figure 3**). AS-OCT allows serial monitoring of inflammatory nodules and synechiae over time, providing a dynamic histopathologic surrogate that informs treatment response and prognosis.

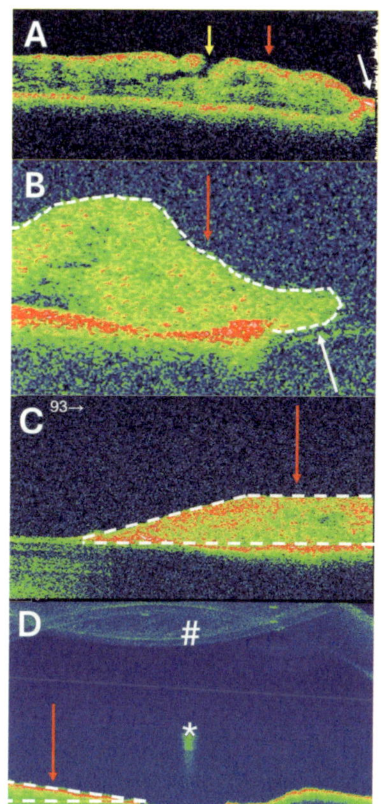

Figure 3.
High-resolution anterior segment optical coherence tomography (AS-OCT) imaging and schematic representation of the iris anatomy. (A) Normal iris structure with notable features: the red arrow indicates an uneven or non-smooth iris surface, the white arrow highlights the hyperreflective extension of the iris pigment epithelium (IPE) at the pupillary ruff, and the yellow arrow points to an iris crypt associated with intrastromal spaces. (B) Koeppe nodule at the pupillary margin: The white dotted line outlines the irregular surface of the iris, while the white arrow shows a gap between the lens capsule and the Koeppe nodule. The hyperreflective signal of the anterior limiting layer is absent in this region, indicating focal disruption. (C) Hyperreflective extension of the anterior limiting layer onto the lens capsule: This extension causes traction on the iris surface, resulting in a smoother appearance (red arrow) and forming an acute angle at the site of adhesion (dashed white lines). (D) Advanced posterior synechiae: The red arrow shows hyperreflective adhesions between the anterior limiting layer of the iris and the lens capsule, forming an acute angle (dashed white lines) at the adhesion site. The asterisk (*) marks a signal saturation artifact, likely caused by high reflectivity from adjacent structures. The hashtag (#) indicates a corneal mirror artifact, reflecting corneal structures into the anterior chamber.

- *Chronic posterior synechiae (PS) formation*: PS develops through the migration of fibromelanocytic cells from the iris's anterior limiting (border) layer onto the lens capsule. AS-OCT captures these hyperreflective adhesions, which are anchored by the lens capsule's robust basement membrane (BM). This intact BM resists degradation by enzymes, inflammatory mediators, or microbial proteases [15–17].

    o *Irreversibility*: Once established, PS undergoes fibrotic collagen deposition. This process manifests on AS-OCT as dense, hyperreflective bands that often necessitate mechanical intervention (by medicines or surgical methods) since anti-inflammatory treatments alone are insufficient for reversing mature adhesions (**Figure 4**).

- *Koeppe nodules and anterior limiting layer disruption*: AS-OCT identifies focal loss of the anterior limiting layer's hyperreflective signal adjacent to Koeppe nodules, suggesting a breakdown of the structural barrier that normally restricts inflammatory cell migration. This disruption may permit outpouching of cellular infiltration from the iris border, reflecting an active inflammatory state and a localized loss of immune privilege. This feature resolved post-corticosteroid therapy (**Figure 4**), underscoring AS-OCT's utility in monitoring granulomatous activity [18]. AS-OCT can visualize Busacca nodules as iris stromal lesions; however, specific imaging reports remain limited in the literature, whereas Berlin nodules, located at the iridocorneal angle, have been described as hyporeflective with hyperreflective borders and have shown regression following corticosteroid therapy [19].

    o *Reversibility*: In contrast to PS, these nodules typically resolve with corticosteroid treatment. As the inflammation subsides, AS-OCT demonstrates a return to normal continuity of the anterior limiting layer.

- *Lens capsule integrity*: The basement membrane (BM) of the lens capsule acts as both a physical barrier and an immunological checkpoint by attracting regulatory T-cells (Tregs) and limiting the migration of inflammatory cells into the lens substance, thus preserving its clarity even in severe anterior segment inflammatory conditions, such as endophthalmitis or advanced uveitis [20]. AS-OCT imaging confirms that the lens capsule's BM remains structurally intact despite adjacent inflammation. Additionally, AS-OCT observations revealing a distinct gap between Koeppe's granulomas and the lens capsule (**Figure 3B**, white arrow, and **Figure 4A**) further support this immune regulatory function [16, 18, 21].

AS-OCT is revolutionizing uveitis management by enabling early detection of pre-fibrotic posterior synechiae, which facilitates timely intervention before irreversible fibrosis sets in. Assessment of anterior limiting layer integrity presents a promising imaging biomarker, potentially aiding in the prediction of recurrent granulomatous inflammation. Furthermore, basement membrane–preserving agents, such as TIMP-3 analogs, may offer targeted therapeutic strategies by inhibiting pathological cellular migration [22]. Despite current gaps in correlating AS-OCT findings with iris biopsy data, emerging 4D AS-OCT technology and AI-driven analysis hold significant promise for real-time tracking of immune cell movement and for distinguishing between reversible and irreversible adhesions (**Figure 4**), thereby paving the way for more personalized and effective clinical interventions.

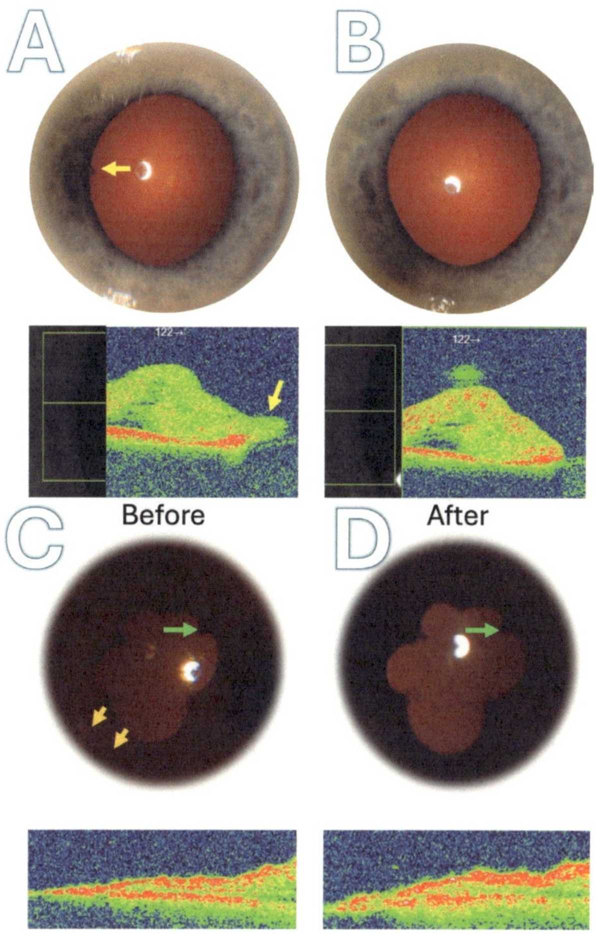

Figure 4.
Comparison of Koeppe nodules and posterior synechiae (PS) Before and After Treatment. (A–B) Slit-lamp and anterior segment optical coherence tomography (AS-OCT) images of a Koeppe nodule at the pupillary margin (yellow arrow) before (A) and after (B) one month of corticosteroid treatment. AS-OCT shows resolution of the hyperreflective lesion at the iris margin, consistent with the reversibility of Koeppe nodules following anti-inflammatory therapy. (C–D) Slit-lamp and AS-OCT images of posterior synechiae (PS) before (C) and after (D) one month of combined corticosteroid and mydriatic eyedrop therapy. Yellow arrows in (C) indicate granulomatous keratic precipitates (KPs), and green arrows mark iris-lens adhesions. Resolution of KPs on slit-lamp examination indicates reduced intraocular inflammation. AS-OCT confirms the persistence of PS, which, if extensive, increases the risk of iris bombe. When pharmacologic dilation does not resolve synechiae, surgical intervention such as synechiolysis or peripheral iridotomy may be considered.

3.2 Corneal changes and keratic precipitates (KPs)

AS-OCT is instrumental in evaluating corneal alterations and KP morphology [23] in uveitis. Larger, more reflective KPs with pronounced posterior shadowing are typically associated with granulomatous uveitis, whereas smaller, less reflective KPs without significant shadowing suggest non-granulomatous inflammation:

- *Non-granulomatous uveitis*: Non-granulomatous KPs are smaller in size compared to granulomatous KPs, typically stellate or coin-shaped, and measure between 5 and 50 μm on AS-OCT, and uniformly hyperreflective with less significant posterior shadowing. The cellular composition includes mainly lymphocytes and neutrophils, reflecting acute, non-granulomatous inflammation [24]. Corneal edema (**Figure 5E**) manifests as stromal thickening and hyperreflectivity due to corneal endothelial dysfunction [25, 26].

- *Granulomatous uveitis*: Hemispheric hyperreflective KPs (50–150 μm) with posterior shadowing (**Figure 5B** and **C**) are typical of sarcoidosis or tuberculosis. These KPs are composed primarily of macrophages, epithelioid cells, and multinucleated giant cells [26].

- *Band keratopathy*: Band keratopathy is a degenerative corneal condition characterized by fine, reflective calcium deposits that typically localize in the subepithelial space, Bowman's layer, and anterior stroma. On AS-OCT, these deposits

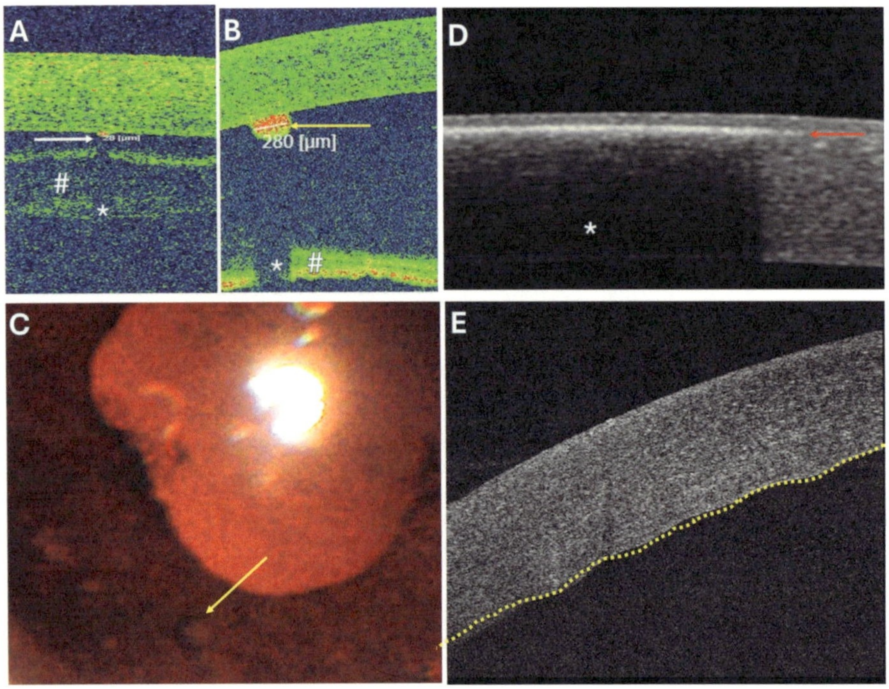

Figure 5.
Anterior segment optical coherence tomography (AS-OCT) imaging of hyperreflective keratic precipitates (KPs), band keratopathy, and corneal edema. (A) Anterior segment optical coherence tomography (AS-OCT) image showing a small non-granulomatous keratic precipitate (KP) on the corneal endothelium (white arrow), measuring 28 μm. The asterisk (*) indicates posterior shadowing caused by the KP, while the hashtag (#) represents an iris mirror artifact, a common imaging phenomenon where the iris structure is reflected within the anterior chamber. (B) AS-OCT image depicting a large globular granulomatous KP (yellow arrow) on the corneal endothelium, measuring 280 μm. Significant posterior shadowing (*) and an iris mirror artifact (#) are visible, consistent with granulomatous inflammation. (C) Slit-lamp photograph correlating with AS-OCT findings, showing a large globular granulomatous KP (yellow arrow) on the corneal endothelium. This image highlights the clinical appearance of granulomatous uveitis. (D) AS-OCT image demonstrating corneal band keratopathy (red arrow), where hyperreflective deposits are seen in the anterior cornea, involving the subepithelial zone, Bowman's layer, and superficial stroma. The asterisk (*) denotes posterior shadowing caused by these calcium deposits. E: AS-OCT image showing corneal stromal edema with Descemet's membrane (DM) folds (outlined by the yellow dotted line). This indicates fluid accumulation within the stroma, often associated with corneal endothelial dysfunction and/or active inflammation in uveitis.

appear as hyperreflective bands with or without posterior shadowing, often correlating with chronic inflammation (**Figure 5D**) [27, 28].

Figure 5 illustrates these key corneal changes, including band keratopathy, KPs, and stromal edema in granulomatous and non-granulomatous uveitis.

3.3 Anterior chamber inflammation quantification

AS-OCT objectively quantifies AC inflammation by detecting hyperreflective dots and flare [29]:

- *Hyperreflective dots*: The Standardization of Uveitis Nomenclature (SUN) Working Group established this grading scheme to standardize the assessment of AC inflammation by quantifying the number of cells observed in a 1 × 1 mm slit beam (magnification x16) field during SLE [30]. AS-OCT imaging detects inflammatory cells as hyperreflective dots within the AC (**Figure 6**). The magnification scale shown in AS-OCT systems like the Topcon Triton corresponds to real dimensions in micrometers, as the software provides direct caliper measurements rather than conventional magnification levels seen in optical microscopy. Studies have demonstrated a strong correlation between the number of these hyperreflective dots and the SUN grading, validating AS-OCT as a reliable tool for assessing AC inflammation [31–33]. Advancements in image analysis algorithms have enabled automated detection and quantification of hyperreflective dots on AS-OCT images. These technologies can identify subclinical inflammation that may not be detected during SLEs, offering a more objective and reproducible assessment of AC inflammation [11, 34, 35]. For a detailed comparison of SUN grading and corresponding AS-OCT findings, see **Table 3**. **Figure 6** shows representative AS-OCT images of hyperreflective dots used in AC inflammation grading.

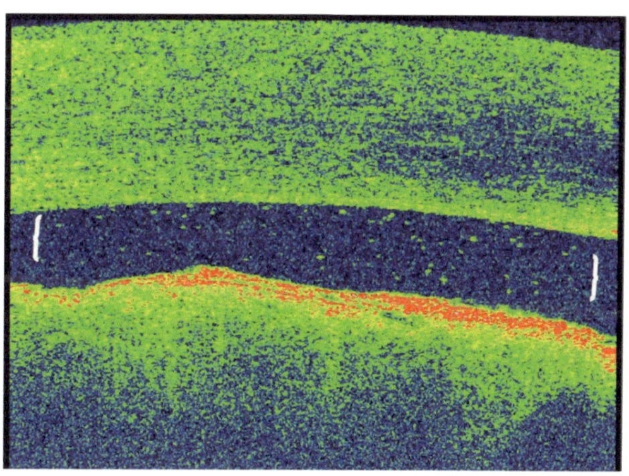

Figure 6.
AS-OCT imaging of hyperreflective dots in the anterior chamber. This AS-OCT image shows hyperreflective dots (enclosed within white brackets {}) in the anterior chamber (AC), localized to the inferior part of the AC. These dots represent red blood cells (RBCs) and AC hemorrhage, but AS-OCT cannot differentiate between cell types, pigments, or debris. The inability to distinguish these elements highlights a limitation of AS-OCT in identifying the exact nature of hyperreflective particles in the AC. This image underscores the utility of AS-OCT in detecting AC abnormalities while emphasizing its diagnostic limitations in cellular differentiation.

SUN grade	Cells per 1 × 1 mm slit beam field	AS-OCT findings
0	<1 cell	No or rare hyperreflective dots
0.5+	1–5 cells	Few isolated hyperreflective dots
1+	6–15 cells	Scattered hyperreflective dots
2+	16–25 cells	Moderate number of hyperreflective dots
3+	26–50 cells	Dense clustering of hyperreflective dots
4+	50 cells	Extensive, confluent hyperreflective signals

Table 3.
Comparison of standardization of uveitis nomenclature (SUN) classification and AS-OCT findings for anterior chamber cells.

- *Aqueous-to-air relative intensity index*: Reflects aqueous flare intensity and correlates with laser flare photometry ($p < 0.0001$) [2, 36, 37].

- *Differentiating cell types*: Recent advances have demonstrated the potential for AS-OCT to differentiate between inflammatory cells and pigment granules based on particle size and reflectivity [38]. Fourier-domain AS-OCT has also shown potential in distinguishing polymorphonuclear cells from mononuclear cells based on axial size and reflectivity characteristics [39]. While these findings are promising, more validation is needed before AS-OCT can reliably characterize specific immune cell subtypes (**Figure 6**).

While AS-OCT reliably detects inflammatory cells, its ability to quantify flare remains limited due to light scattering artifacts. LFP remains the gold standard for flare assessment.

3.4 Iris and pupillary changes

AS-OCT provides high-resolution imaging of iris structures to differentiate uveitic subtypes:

- *Granulomatous uveitis*: Koeppe, Busacca, and Berlin nodules appear as hyperreflective lesions on AS-OCT [18, 19]. In Koeppe nodules, a lack of signal from the anterior limiting layer has been documented during the active inflammatory phase [18]. In the non-active phase, hyperreflective dots typically disappear or become sparse on AS-OCT, reflecting clinical resolution of intraocular inflammation (**Figure 4B**). Residual particles may persist in some cases as non-cellular debris or pigment granules [40].

- *Fuchs' uveitis syndrome (FUS):* In FUS, diffuse iris stromal thinning with smooth surface architecture is observed [41], along with wider iridocorneal angles compared to Posner-Schlossman syndrome (PSS) [42].

- *Crystalline deposits:* Iris crystals are a rare clinical finding typically associated with chronic anterior uveitis (CAU), particularly in Fuchs' uveitis and idiopathic chronic iridocyclitis. However, AS-OCT images of these findings remain limited in the literature and were not available in our clinical series. These crystalline deposits are typically composed of cholesterol or calcium deposits, which can be observed on the iris surface, corneal endothelium, and anterior lens capsule [40]. AS-OCT effectively identifies these crystals as hyperreflective deposits in these locations. Long-term monitoring indicates that these deposits are typically stable but may become dislodged or reabsorbed following intraocular surgery or trauma [40, 43].

3.5 Angle assessment and glaucoma mechanisms

AS-OCT plays a pivotal role in evaluating the anterior chamber angle (ACA) and detecting glaucoma-related changes:

- *Steroid-induced ocular hypertension*:

Chronic corticosteroid use can lead to the accumulation of extracellular matrix components, such as glycosaminoglycans, within the trabecular meshwork (TM), increasing outflow resistance and causing a rise in intraocular pressure (IOP). AS-OCT has shown that eyes with steroid-induced ocular hypertension exhibit a significantly reduced TM height, reflecting structural compromise at the outflow pathway [44]. Importantly, this condition occurs with an open iridocorneal angle, distinguishing it from secondary angle-closure glaucoma seen in uveitic eyes, where posterior synechiae (PS) or peripheral anterior synechiae (PAS) lead to mechanical angle closure. AS-OCT thus helps differentiate between these pathophysiologic mechanisms by visualizing angle configuration, TM height, and synechial adhesions [45].

- *Trabeculitis:*

Localized hyperreflective regions within the TM suggest inflammatory trabeculitis, often associated with herpetic [46], cytomegalovirus (CMV)-related uveitis [47], or PSS [48]. It is important to note that trabeculitis diagnosis is often presumptive and requires clinical correlation, as AS-OCT findings are nonspecific and can mimic other causes of TM edema. TM edema may contribute to IOP elevation by obstructing aqueous outflow. These findings support the use of anti-inflammatory therapies to reduce TM edema and improve IOP control in PSS.

- *Uveitis-glaucoma-hyphema (UGH) syndrome*:

UGH syndrome is associated with chronic inflammation, hemorrhage, or elevated IOP (see Section 3.6) [49].

- *Peripheral anterior synechiae (PAS)*:

On AS-OCT, PAS appear as hyperreflective bands of iris tissue extending anteriorly to attach to the angle's wall, often causing obliteration of the angle recess. Unlike appositional angle closure, which shows contact without structural change (**Figure 7C**), PAS exhibits a broad-based, fixed adhesion with no visible cleft between the iris and corneoscleral wall. These synechiae often distort normal angle anatomy and may appear as bridging structures, sometimes with underlying angle pigmentation or irregularity. AS-OCT enables non-contact, high-resolution imaging useful in cases where gonioscopy is difficult—such as in corneal edema, active uveitis, or pediatric patients—and supports the evaluation of extent, quadrant distribution, and potential

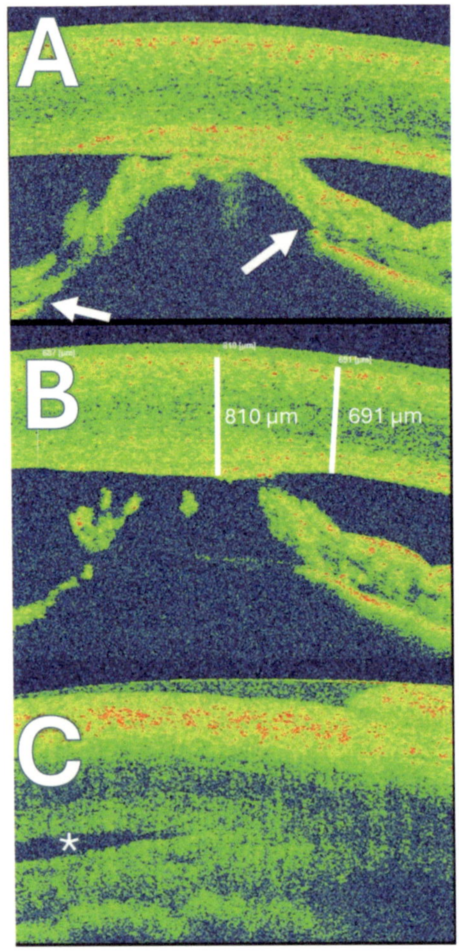

Figure 7.
AS-OCT imaging of post-cataract surgery iatrogenic iridocorneal adhesion. (A) AS-OCT image illustrating a post-cataract surgery iatrogenic iridocorneal adhesion. The adhesion is characterized by disruption of the iris pigment epithelium (IPE) (indicated by white arrows). Adjacent corneal stromal thickening is marked with a dashed yellow outline, highlighting localized signal changes. (B) High-resolution AS-OCT image showing measurements of corneal thickness adjacent to the adhesion (810 µm and 691 µm). The AS-OCT image shows localized corneal stromal edema with increased thickness and hyperreflectivity, consistent with structural remodeling adjacent to the adhesion. This stromal edema may result from chronic low-grade inflammation, impaired endothelial function adjacent to the adhesion, or mechanical traction from fibrotic synechiae disrupting corneal hydration. Additionally, overproduction of extracellular matrix during healing, infiltration of inflammatory cells from the iris, or focal regeneration of iris pigment epithelial cell islands entrapped in the posterior stroma may contribute to localized tissue remodeling. (C) AS-OCT image depicting open anterior chamber angle (*) peripheral to the adhesion. The absence of hyperreflective bridging tissue and layers over the angle or corneal periphery and the preservation of the angle recess indicates that the adhesion is not caused by migratory traction from fibromelanocytic cells extending over these areas, distinguishing it from peripheral anterior synechiae (PAS).

angle obstruction in uveitic or angle-closure glaucoma. While AS-OCT may not always differentiate chronic PAS from early or partial synechiae, its ability to document angle changes objectively enhances clinical decision-making and follow-up in anterior segment pathology [50, 51]. AS-OCT detection of PAS or angle narrowing in uveitis should prompt early glaucoma risk assessment and possible gonioscopic confirmation. Detection of extensive PAS on AS-OCT should prompt consideration of aggressive IOP management and potential surgical intervention to prevent glaucomatous damage.

3.6 Lens and cataract evaluation

AS-OCT provides valuable insights into cataract morphology and anterior segment integrity, aiding in preoperative planning and postoperative management of uveitic eyes undergoing cataract surgery. By differentiating types of cataracts and identifying complex presentations such as phacolytic glaucoma, phacoantigenic, or phacoanaphylactic conditions in the presence of uveitis background, AS-OCT enhances surgical outcomes and patient care.

- *Preoperative assessment with AS-OCT*
    - AS-OCT plays a crucial role in preoperative assessment by providing detailed images of the anterior segment, which can guide treatment decisions in uveitic eyes undergoing cataract surgery.
    - *Cataract type characterization*: AS-OCT helps differentiate between various cataract types, such as posterior polar cataracts and posterior subcapsular cataracts (PSC), by evaluating the morphology of lens opacities. For example, posterior polar cataracts often involve a central opacity in the posterior capsule, while PSCs are characterized by opacities in the posterior subcapsular region of the lens [52].
    - *Capsule integrity*: AS-OCT assesses the integrity of the posterior capsule, which is essential for surgical planning. It helps identify posterior capsular defects in traumatic and posterior polar cataracts, and evaluates residual capsular support scenarios involving IOL opacification, aphakia in young uveitic patients, or prior to secondary IOL implantation [53].
    - *Inflammatory vs. steroid-induced cataracts*: AS-OCT can distinguish between inflammatory cataracts and steroid-induced cataracts. Inflammatory cataracts typically exhibit lens opacities, capsular thickening, and pericapsular inflammatory membranes, whereas steroid-induced cataracts usually present as classic posterior subcapsular opacities without adjacent inflammatory features [54].
    - *Phacolytic glaucoma*: AS-OCT aids in detecting lamellar separation and cortical liquefaction, particularly in phacolytic glaucoma, helping differentiate between lens-induced inflammation and primary intraocular inflammation. This condition is characterized by the leakage of high-molecular-weight lens proteins through an intact lens capsule, leading to trabecular meshwork obstruction and secondary open-angle glaucoma [47, 55].
- *Postoperative assessment with AS-OCT*

    Postoperatively, AS-OCT is useful for differentiating inflammatory membranes from true IOL material degradation and opacifications. This distinction is crucial for managing postoperative complications and ensuring optimal IOL function.

- *Inflammatory membranes vs. IOL opacifications*: AS-OCT can identify inflammatory membranes, which may form in response to uveitis or surgical trauma, and distinguish them from IOL opacifications such as calcifications [56].

Inflammatory membranes typically appear as hyperreflective layers anterior to the IOL, whereas IOL opacifications demonstrate distinct internal reflectivity patterns depending on their composition [57–59]. AS-OCT may help prevent unnecessary YAG laser procedures by accurately identifying these entities.

- *IOL position*: AS-OCT evaluates the position of the IOL and its interaction with surrounding ocular structures, helping to detect malposition or contact with the iris, which can lead to complications like UGH syndrome [49].

3.7 Anterior vitreous inflammation

The SUN Working Group has established a grading system for vitreous haze, which assesses the clarity of the ocular fundus during examination. AS-OCT was utilized to quantify anterior vitreous cells in cases of intermediate uveitis. The findings demonstrated a significant correlation between AS-OCT measurements and SUN vitreous haze grades ($p < 0.001$), suggesting that AS-OCT can serve as an objective tool to assess vitreous inflammation. This approach has the potential to reduce interobserver variability inherent in manual grading methods; however, further validation is necessary to fully establish its clinical utility [60].

- *Vitreous assessment: Differentiating Vitreoretinal Lymphoma (VRL) from Uveitis-associated Vitritis*

  Radiomics is an emerging AI technique that extracts texture, intensity, and shape-based features from imaging datasets. When applied to AS-OCT, it may help differentiate VRL from inflammatory vitritis based on distinct cellular and haze patterns. In VRL, AS-OCT reveals non-clumped, sheet-like cellular arrangements in the anterior vitreous. These cells are typically larger and more isolated compared to the densely packed inflammatory cells in uveitis. While representative AS-OCT images of VRL patterns were not available in our clinical archive, these patterns are well-described in the literature. The 'aurora borealis' configuration refers to linear cellular alignment along vitreous fibrils, whereas the 'string of pearls' denotes clustered hyperreflective foci arranged in chains. In contrast, inflammatory vitritis typically appears as a diffuse, amorphous haze without structured organization. These features aid in distinguishing VRL from uveitis-associated vitritis. However, the current approach is limited by manual cell counting, retrospective study designs, small sample sizes, and a lack of comparison with established diagnostic markers [61]. Future studies should focus on prospective validation and integration with cytopathologic markers to refine non-invasive diagnostic criteria for VRL.

4. Differentiating uveitis subtypes and associated conditions

4.1 Granulomatous vs. non-granulomatous uveitis

AS-OCT distinguishes granulomatous from non-granulomatous uveitis based on distinct anterior segment features, including iris nodules, KP morphology, and corneal changes:

- *Granulomatous*:
    - *KP morphology*: See above [25, 26, 50].
    - *Iris granulomas*: AS-OCT can also visualize iris nodules, which are indicative of granulomatous inflammation. These granulomas appear as distinct, hyper-reflective lesions on the iris surface [3, 62].
- *Non-granulomatous*:
    - *KP morphology*: See above [26].
    - *Corneal Stromal Edema*: Stromal edema due to endothelial dysfunction is a common feature in non-granulomatous uveitis. This edema can be visualized as increased corneal thickness and signal changes on AS-OCT, indicating compromised corneal endothelial function. In corneal stromal edema, AS-OCT reveals increased corneal thickness with disruption of the normal stromal lamellar pattern. The reflectivity becomes heterogeneous or reduced in areas due to interlamellar fluid accumulation and light scattering, often resulting in blurring of stromal layers and posterior signal attenuation [26, 63].

4.2 Infectious uveitis

AS-OCT identifies specific patterns in infectious uveitis subtypes:

- *Herpetic keratouveitis*: AS-OCT detects retrocorneal plaques, TM hyperreflectivity (trabeculitis), iris stromal atrophy (**Figure 8**), and corneal stromal edema [46, 64, 65].
- *CMV uveitis:* CMV anterior uveitis often presents with coin-shaped KPs that appear as discrete, highly reflective lesions on AS-OCT. These differ from the irregular, retrocorneal deposits typically seen in HSV/VZV uveitis [47].
- *Monkeypox (Mpox):* In Mpox-associated uveitis, AS-OCT has revealed sub-endothelial deposits and stromal edema, findings that may help distinguish it from herpetic or idiopathic etiologies [66].
- *Rubella uveitis*: Reduced iris stromal thickness and atrophy compared to CMV [67].
- *Tuberculosis/Leprosy*: Nodular iris/angle lesions; AS-OCT can track granuloma regression [50, 62].
- *Syphilis*: In syphilitic uveitis, AS-OCT may identify iris masses with hyporeflective rims, potentially representing granulomatous nodules. These nodules typically regress following systemic penicillin therapy [68, 69].

4.3 Masquerade syndromes

AS-OCT aids in detecting non-inflammatory conditions mimicking uveitis, such as neoplasms, drug-induced toxicities, or intraocular foreign bodies (IOFBs):

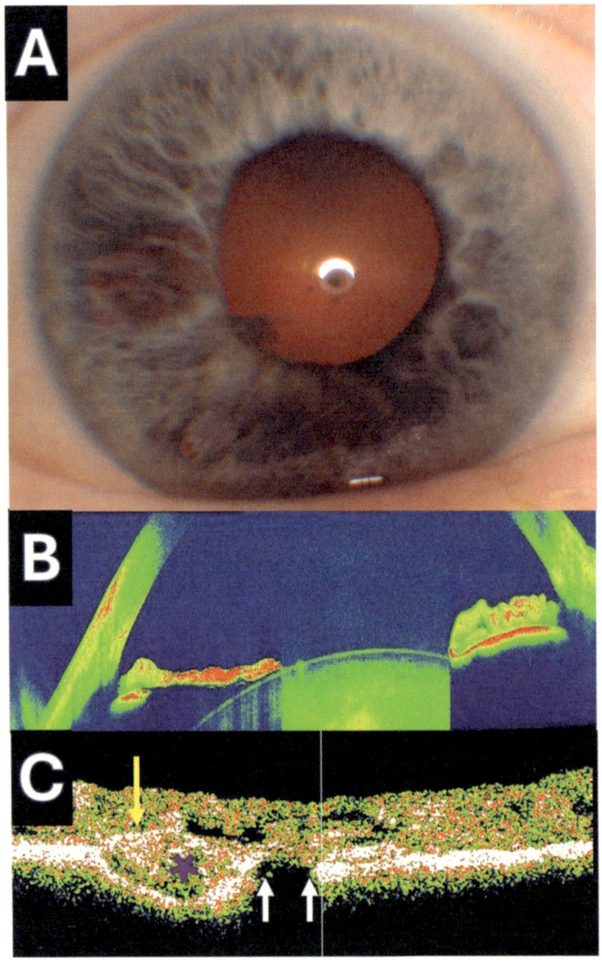

Figure 8.
AS-OCT and clinical findings in herpetic (HSV-1) anterior uveitis. (A) Slit-lamp photograph showing iris stromal atrophy with transillumination and depigmentation, characteristic of herpetic anterior uveitis. (B) AS-OCT image demonstrating structural changes in the iris, including stromal thinning and significant atrophy. (C) High-resolution color-enhanced AS-OCT highlighting disruption of the posterior pigment epithelium of the iris (white arrows), separation of the anterior (yellow arrow) and posterior pigmented epithelium (purple asterisk), and areas of iris smoothing with stromal atrophy.

- *Drug toxicity*: AS-OCT reveals characteristic changes such as iris stromal thinning, loss of pigment epithelium, and posterior concavity. These findings are consistent with the clinical presentation of bilateral acute iris transillumination (BAIT) in fluoroquinolone-associated irits. Such changes have been associated with certain antiviral agents (e.g., cidofovir) and fluoroquinolones (e.g., moxifloxacin) [70, 71].

- *Iris stromal cysts*: Confirms cyst size regression and corneal endothelial cell loss, enabling non-invasive monitoring [72].

- *Neoplasms:*

- *Diffuse anterior retinoblastoma (Rb)*: AS-OCT identifies progressive tumor growth and stromal invasion in Rb [73].

- *Metastatic iris tumors*: AS-OCT provides non-invasive assessment of iris metastases from primary tumors such as lung, breast, melanoma, prostate, gastrointestinal, and renal carcinomas. Characteristic features include nodular or diffuse iris thickening with disrupted stromal architecture [74–76]. These imaging findings can guide diagnostic interventions such as fine needle aspiration biopsy and monitor response to local radiotherapy or systemic chemotherapy. Importantly, iris metastases may be the first manifestation of an undiagnosed systemic malignancy, making AS-OCT a critical tool in early diagnosis. Its non-invasive nature, combined with detailed structural visualization, supports its integration into routine evaluation of atypical iris lesions in patients with known or suspected malignancy [77].

- *Intraocular foreign bodies (IOFBs):* AS-OCT aids in differentiating IOFBs based on their composition. Metallic foreign bodies typically appear as hyperreflective structures on AS-OCT, often accompanied by a mirror effect or posterior shadowing due to their high density [78]. Organic materials, such as wood or vegetative matter, may present as hyperreflective structures with shadowing; however, their appearance can vary, and in some cases, they may not be easily detectable, especially if they are small or have similar reflectivity to surrounding tissues. AS-OCT enables detection of small or low-density foreign bodies—such as organic (vegetal) material—that may be radiolucent and thus undetectable by conventional X-ray or CT. These objects typically appear as well-defined, hyperreflective lesions with posterior shadowing or localized disruption of adjacent tissue planes [79, 80]. Insect wing corneal foreign bodies, may show hyperreflective, well-delineated structures in AS-OCT. The imaging can aid in differentiating these from as hyperreflective lesions like uveal prolapse or pigmented ocular surface tumors [81]. Glass IOFBs typically lack internal reflectivity and exhibit sharp borders, making them readily identifiable on AS-OCT [78]. By analyzing these reflectivity patterns, AS-OCT assists clinicians in accurately identifying the nature of IOFBs, thereby informing appropriate management strategies and potentially reducing unnecessary interventions.

- *Post-surgical infections*: Postoperative infections can mimic sterile intraocular inflammation, making accurate diagnosis challenging. AS-OCT enhances anterior segment structural visualization by providing high-resolution, cross-sectional images of the corneal wound site and adjacent sclera. In cases of late-onset fungal tunnel infections, AS-OCT can reveal dense, localized hyperreflective lesions that extend from the corneal incision into the scleral tunnel, which may be missed on SLE alone. This imaging feature helps differentiate infectious from non-infectious etiologies and can prompt timely initiation of antifungal therapy, as in reported cases where presumed recurrent uveitis was ultimately diagnosed as a fungal infection based on AS-OCT findings [82].

- *Dynamic mobile pigment clumps*: Dynamic mobile pigment clumps, often observed in patients reporting entoptic phenomena, can resemble other hyperreflective intraocular structures such as inflammatory cells, fibrin, or neoplastic aggregates. AS-OCT aids in distinguishing these entities by allowing real-time, cross-sectional visualization of the anterior chamber. Pigment clumps typically appear as discrete, highly reflective particles with no posterior shadowing and are freely mobile in response to blinking or eye movements, which can be appreciated during dynamic scanning. In contrast, inflammatory cells tend to be more diffuse, while malignant cells (e.g., in VRL) form clumps or sheets with persistent structure and positional stability. Recognizing these distinctions on AS-OCT helps avoid unnecessary immunosuppression or biopsy [83].

AS-OCT may differentiate benign from malignant iris or conjunctival lesions based on epithelial thickness, stromal invasion, and the transition zone with underlying structures, helping to distinguish inflammatory nodules from neoplastic processes. Posterior segment OCT can reveal features atypical for uveitis, such as subretinal infiltrates, outer retinal atrophy, or hyperreflective clumps in the vitreous and retina, which are suggestive of lymphoma or leukemia rather than true inflammation. These structural findings, especially when unaccompanied by classic signs of inflammation like vascular leakage, should prompt consideration of masquerade syndromes and guide further diagnostic evaluation through multimodal imaging and cytopathologic confirmation.

4.4 Pediatric uveitis

AS-OCT provides a non-contact imaging alternative for pediatric patients with poor slit-lamp compliance [84]:

- Diagnostic Advantages:
  - *Non-contact, rapid imaging*: Well-tolerated by children (median time < 10 minutes; acceptability ≥8.5/10) [85].
  - *Objective inflammation assessment*: Correlates with SUN grading (92% sensitivity, 86% specificity) [85, 86].
  - *Clinical applications*: AS-OCT plays a crucial role in detecting hyperreflective aqueous cells, posterior synechiae, and band keratopathy, and it can resolve ambiguous cases involving pearl-like highly reflective masses attached to the posterior cornea. These masses might represent inflammatory or fibrotic deposits that resolve with steroid therapy. These capabilities highlight AS-OCT's utility in managing complex anterior segment pathologies [87].
- *JIA-associated uveitis:*
  - *AS-OCT findings*: Band keratopathy (hyperreflective calcific deposits), posterior synechiae, and hyperreflective aqueous cells.
  - *Clinical utility*: Interpretation of pediatric AS-OCT images remains limited by the absence of age-stratified normative databases, particularly for AC cell counts and iris reflectivity. The *UVESCREEN1* study (ClinicalTrials.gov Identifier: NCT05984758), with an anticipated study completion date of October 2026, is an ongoing, pioneering 12-month randomized controlled trial designed to evaluate the feasibility and clinical effectiveness of imaging-based uveitis

screening using AS-OCT compared to traditional SLE in children with Juvenile Idiopathic Arthritis (JIA). The study aimed at validating AS-OCT-based screening protocols in pediatric anterior uveitis may establish AS-OCT as a triage or follow-up tool in resource-limited or non-slit-lamp-accessible settings [88].

While OCT devices are more expensive than slit-lamp biomicroscopes, in many developed healthcare systems—including smaller cities and non-tertiary centers—the main challenge is not acquiring the device, but ensuring the availability of skilled personnel to perform and interpret slit-lamp examinations. As OCT systems become more portable and cost-effective, their integration into primary and secondary care—even in smaller urban centers—is increasingly feasible.

This study involves 80 children aged 2–12 years who were diagnosed with JIA within the preceding year. The primary focus is on assessing feasibility metrics, clinical outcomes, quality-of-life evaluations, and resource utilization [88].

While SLEs are crucial for assessing uveitis, they can be uncomfortable for photosensitive patients due to the high-intensity light used. In contrast, OCT imaging offers a more tolerable alternative, utilizing low-intensity laser light that minimizes discomfort and photophobia, making it an attractive option for managing uveitis in sensitive patients. While children who are uncooperative during SLEs may also present challenges during AS-OCT imaging, the rapid, non-contact nature of AS-OCT, combined with automated alignment and emerging robotic systems, can make it more feasible for pediatric patients. Even in partially cooperative patients, brief stillness is often sufficient for image capture, unlike slit-lamp examination, which requires prolonged fixation and clinician interaction. In this context, AS-OCT serves as a valuable adjunct for screening or documentation in children and uncooperative patients where traditional exams may be impractical.

Moreover, the feasibility of AS-OCT screening by non-ophthalmologists, utilizing AI, could potentially broaden access to uveitis screening. Preliminary results have demonstrated high sensitivity and specificity of AS-OCT in detecting anterior uveitis among pediatric patients [85, 86]. The modality has been well-tolerated [85, 86], feasible with excellent reliability [89]; however, concerns have been raised regarding inter-device [90] and inter-operator variability [91], as well as a higher rate of false-positive results than SLE [90]. The findings from UVESCREEN1 are expected to be instrumental in guiding future research and informing clinical guidelines on the use of imaging-based modalities for uveitis screening in pediatric populations. Addressing key challenges such as standardizing imaging protocols, minimizing inter-device and inter-operator variability, and refining AI algorithms to reduce false-positive rates will be essential for successful integration of AS-OCT into routine clinical workflows. Uniform image acquisition strategies and validated grading platforms can improve reproducibility, while AI-enhanced interpretation holds potential for expanding access beyond tertiary care centers. These efforts will ensure AS-OCT's diagnostic utility is consistent, scalable, and clinically actionable.

- *Blau syndrome:*

Blau syndrome (BS), a rare autoinflammatory disorder, presents unique challenges in managing ocular inflammation. While several AS-OCT findings such as keratic precipitates and anterior chamber cells are common to many forms of uveitis, certain entities may exhibit distinctive features. Blau syndrome—a rare autoinflammatory granulomatous disease—can present with iris stromal thickening, large granulomatous KPs, and nodular anterior segment lesions that are likely to appear as hyperreflective masses on AS-OCT. These findings, when combined with systemic signs such as arthritis and dermatitis, can help differentiate Blau syndrome from other granulomatous uveitides like sarcoidosis or tuberculosis.

  - *AS-OCT findings*: Hyperreflective aqueous humor cells, posterior synechiae, and corneal band keratopathy [92].

- *Challenges*:

  - *False positives*: Normative hyperreflective spots within the AC of healthy children (76% of eyes) complicate inflammation detection [93]. Normative hyperreflective spots observed on AS-OCT in pediatric patients are non-cellular reflections that can mimic inflammation.

  - *Device variability*: Heidelberg Spectralis OCT1 underperforms vs. CASIA2 in detecting inflammatory cells [90].

  - *Poor specificity*: AS-OCT scans show high sensitivity but low specificity for sub-clinical inflammation [90], primarily due to physiologic hyperreflectivity [93].

  - *Cooperation issues*: Infants or children who cannot remain still despite non-pharmacological interventions may require sedation or portable devices to obtain accurate imaging. The swift capture of images reduces the time the child needs to remain still, enhancing cooperation and reducing the likelihood of requiring sedation. This requires a rapid imaging to avoid sedation in young children.

  - *Penetration limits*: Inability to visualize PC or CB.

- *Future Directions*:

  - Automated inflammatory cell detection to reduce interobserver bias [94].

  - Robotic tracking and rapid acquisition features help mitigate motion artifacts in pediatric imaging, increasing reliability and reducing sedation requirements.

  - Multimodal integration with SLE and LFP: While true integration of AS-OCT, slit-lamp, and LFP into a single diagnostic unit is currently limited in routine outpatient practice, surgical microscopes with intraoperative OCT (iOCT) represent a practical, commercially available multimodal platform already in use during procedures. Further development of combined anterior segment workstations incorporating OCT, SLE, and flare measurement—supported by AI and standardized reference databases—could significantly enhance reproducibility and clinical accuracy, particularly in pediatric or teleophthalmology settings.

  - Standardized pediatric reference datasets help reduce false positives by defining age-specific normative ranges, guiding clinicians and AI systems to distinguish between normal developmental variations and true inflammatory changes. This contextual interpretation is especially important in young children [93].

4.5 Treatment-related complications

AS-OCT detects complications arising from therapeutic interventions such as steroid-induced ocular hypertension (short trabecular meshwork (TM) height) [44] or inadvertent intralenticular implantation of dexamethasone intravitreal implants [95].

5. Challenges in AS-OCT imaging for uveitis

AS-OCT has revolutionized anterior segment imaging in uveitis but faces significant technical and clinical limitations that impede its full diagnostic potential. While AS-OCT is a valuable tool for assessing anterior chamber inflammation, its sensitivity in detecting cells can be affected by factors such as media opacities and image quality. It is noteworthy that AS-OCT may not detect all inflammatory cells, especially in cases with low-grade inflammation or poor image quality. Although hyperreflective dots on AS-OCT are presumed to represent inflammatory cells, this remains unverified due to the absence of cytologic correlation in most studies. They may also include pigment, debris, or imaging artifacts. Motion artifacts, poor fixation, and shadowing

Aspect	Advantages	Disadvantages	Solutions/future perspectives
Anterior segment imaging	Non-invasive, high-resolution imaging of cornea, anterior chamber, and angle structures.	Limited penetration depth; cannot visualize posterior chamber (PC), pars plana (PP), or ciliary body (CB). Limited field of view, it is affected by anatomical factors.	Use contact lens-based mirror OCT systems to extend imaging to the PC, CB, and PP.
Detection of inflammatory cells	Objective detection of hyperreflective dots indicative of anterior chamber inflammation.	Cannot differentiate between inflammatory cells, pigments, or debris.	Combine radiomics with spectroscopic OCT to differentiate cell types based on molecular and reflectivity-based features.
Quantification of KPs and edema	Enables precise measurement of keratic precipitates (KPs) and corneal edema.	Prone to artifacts such as shadowing, mirror artifacts, and saturation artifacts.	Develop AI-driven artifact suppression algorithms to correct imaging artifacts and improve diagnostic accuracy.
Pediatric applications	Well-tolerated by children; provides objective imaging without requiring slit-lamp cooperation.	Requires sedation or rapid imaging protocols for uncooperative pediatric patients in some cases.	Developing portable devices and optimize imaging protocols for faster robotic acquisition and integrate automated alignment systems for pediatric use.
Clinical monitoring	Allows longitudinal monitoring of anterior segment changes during treatment.	Lack of standardized normative databases for pediatric populations or diverse ethnic groups.	Develop age- and ethnicity-specific normative databases for anterior segment parameters to improve diagnostic reliability.

Table 4.
Advantages, disadvantages, and future perspectives of AS-OCT in uveitis.

from corneal opacities or synechiae can obscure the anterior chamber, resulting in underestimation or misidentification of inflammation. Differences in scan resolution, segmentation algorithms, and user-defined acquisition protocols may lead to inconsistencies in data, posing challenges for cross-study or cross-center comparisons. **Table 4** summarizes its advantages and disadvantages while proposing solutions and future perspectives to overcome these challenges. Below, we outline these challenges, discuss future research directions, and conclude with actionable insights for advancing uveitis care.

5.1 Technical and diagnostic limitations

5.1.1 Artifacts and imaging errors

- *Mirror artifacts:* Corneal or iris reflections obscure iris/angle structures, mimicking pathologies like anterior chamber cysts or adhesions (**Figure 3D, 5A** and **B, and 9B** and **C**).

- *Shadowing*:

  o *Dense KPs/Synechiae*: Block posterior visualization (**Figure 5**).

  o *Eyelash interference*: Creates false shadows.

- *Saturation artifacts*: Hyperreflective surfaces (e.g., tear film) cause signal oversaturation, distorting anatomical details (**Figure 3D**).

- *Specular reflections*: Glare from the pupillary margin or iris surface obscures structural details.

- *Sunray/starburst artifacts:* Scatter creates radial hyperreflective lines, and interferes with tissue signals [96]. The source of this scatter is unknown (**Figure 9**).

- *Volume scattering:* Inflammatory debris or nodules generate diffuse hyperreflectivity, complicating cellular differentiation.

- *Signal loss:*

  o *Media opacity:* Cataracts or corneal edema reduce penetration depth.

  o *Positioning errors/blinking:* Misalignment during acquisition creates gaps in imaging.

- *Y-scan reconstruction errors:* Stitched X-scans misrepresent dynamic iris changes and their configuration, leading to irregular and broken Y-scans.

These artifacts, including the distinctive starburst pattern, are depicted in **Figure 9**.

5.1.2 Device limitations

- *Iris imaging:* Commercial systems lack optimization for the iris layer's analysis, hindering histopathological validation [18].

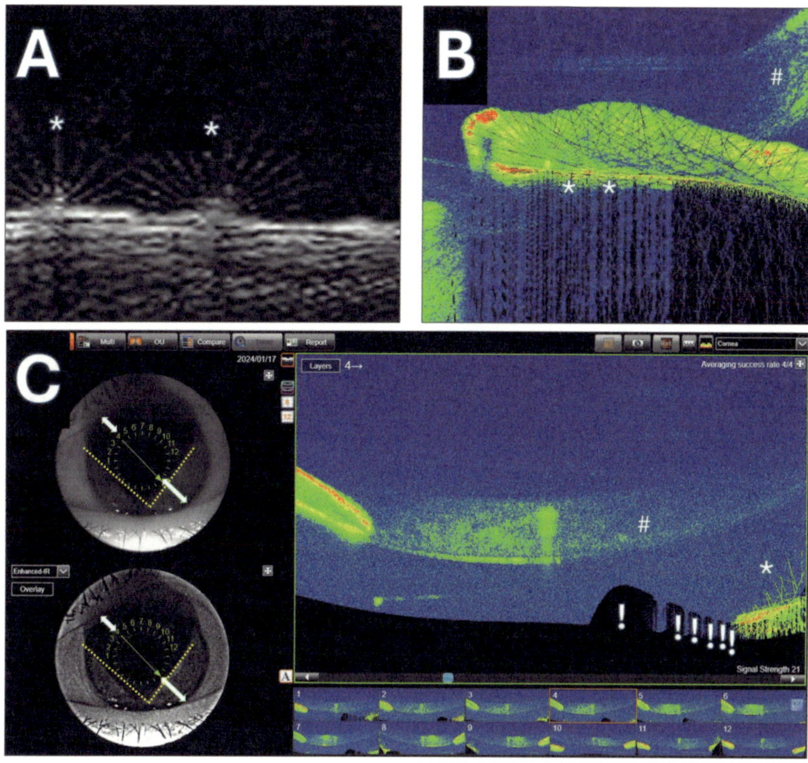

Figure 9.
Sunray/starburst artifacts in anterior segment optical coherence tomography (AS-OCT). (A) Radial hyperreflective lines (asterisks) originating from the iris surface, resembling sunray/starburst artifacts. These artifacts interfere with the visualization of surrounding tissue layers and contribute to signal disruption. (B) High-resolution AS-OCT image showing radial scattering sunray/starburst artifacts (double asterisks) emanating from hyperreflective regions of the iris pigment epithelium (IPE). Volumetric scattering may contribute to these artifacts. The hashtag symbol (#) indicates mirror artifacts originating from the corneal surface. (C) The AS-OCT operator interface demonstrates how the radial scattering sunray/starburst artifacts (asterisk) appear across multiple scan angles. The clock-hour overlay highlights the distribution of scan sections. Misalignment and asymmetric illumination are indicated by solid white arrows, and signal void areas are marked with exclamation points (!). Shadowings (outlined with yellow dashed line) visible in the infrared (IR) photo are caused by suboptimal examination conditions. Are evident, along with shadowing artifacts visible in the infrared (IR) photo, caused by suboptimal examination conditions. The hashtag symbol (#) indicates mirror artifacts from the cornea.

- *Penetration depth:* AS-OCT is limited to a penetration depth of approximately 3 mm, which prevents visualization of deeper structures such as the CB and PC. While AS-OCT excels in high-resolution imaging of anterior segment structures, its ability to detect posterior segment pathology is constrained by this limited depth. For comprehensive ocular assessment, clinicians should supplement AS-OCT with UBM and posterior segment imaging modalities—such as conventional OCT or fundus photography.

- *Device variability:* Variations in axial resolution (CASIA2: 10 μm; Spectralis: 7 μm) and differences in segmentation algorithms contribute to reduced inter-device reproducibility [90, 97]. Compared to the Spectralis HS1, CASIA2 exhibits wider Bland–Altman limits of agreement (+17 to −19 cells vs. +1 to −1 cells), indicating greater variability. The Bland–Altman analysis compares the agreement between two quantitative measurements by plotting the difference versus the average of the two methods. The limits of agreement (mean ± 1.96 SD) indicate the range within which 95% of the differences are expected to lie, providing insight into measurement repeatability. However, CASIA2 compensates for this with significantly higher sensitivity (0.92 vs. 0.17) and a strong association with clinical inflammation grading (correlation coefficient = 12.8, $p = 0.02$). Notably, fluctuations in clinical grade closely parallel changes in image-based cell counts ($r^2 = 0.79$, $p < 0.001$). These findings suggest that despite lower reproducibility, CASIA2's heightened sensitivity and strong clinical alignment make it a valuable tool for monitoring disease activity [90].

Lower reproducibility and higher sensitivity can coexist when a device is capable of detecting extremely small changes or low-level signals that other systems may miss. CASIA2's high axial resolution and contrast sensitivity allow it to register subtle fluctuations in inflammatory activity; however, these small differences may vary slightly between repeated scans due to biological or technical noise. As a result, while the device may show more variability in repeated measurements (lower reproducibility), it remains highly sensitive to early or subclinical disease activity—offering valuable clinical insight that less sensitive devices might overlook.

5.1.3 Diagnostic gaps

Differentiating between sources of hyperreflectivity on AS-OCT—such as inflammatory cells, debris, and fibrosis, presents challenges due to overlapping imaging characteristics. Inflammatory cells often appear as small, discrete, hyperreflective foci within the corneal stroma or AC, potentially representing activated immune cells responding to inflammation [98]. Debris, including lipid or proteinaceous material, manifests as hyperreflective particles, sometimes precursors to more organized deposits like keratic precipitates. Fibrosis presents as more extensive hyperreflective areas associated with structural changes in tissues like the cornea, angle, iris, or lens indicative of scarring processes [99]. Employing multimodal imaging techniques and conducting longitudinal assessments can enhance diagnostic accuracy; however,

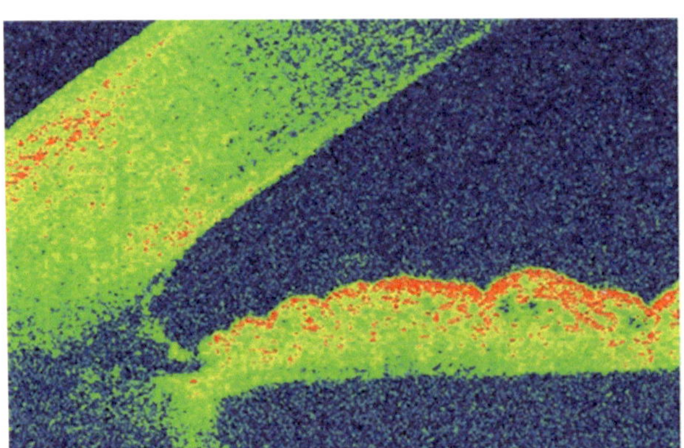

Figure 10.
Iris and angle image in a case of ocular albinism. The AS-OCT image shows the iris and angle region in a patient with ocular albinism. Notably, the hyperreflective signal typically associated with the iris pigment epithelium (IPE) is absent, consistent with the hypopigmentation characteristic of this condition. This case highlights the importance of establishing normative data for iris reflectivity to differentiate normal individual variations from pathological signal differences.

precise differentiation remains complex, highlighting the need for further research and advanced imaging modalities.

- *Inability to differentiate cell types:* AS-OCT cannot reliably distinguish inflammatory cells from pigment or debris [38, 94].

- *Normative data gaps:* There are currently no standardized reference databases for cell grading, iris thickness and reflectivity (**Figure 10**), KP reflectivity, or CB metrics across different age groups or levels of pigmentation [93].

6. Future research directions

Emerging technologies, such as ultrahigh-resolution OCT and AI, hold promise in enhancing the diagnostic capabilities of AS-OCT. Ultrahigh-resolution OCT can provide near-histological imaging of ocular structures, facilitating more precise assessments of inflammatory changes. Concurrently, AI algorithms can assist in the automated detection and quantification of AC cells, offering objective metrics for disease monitoring and treatment efficacy evaluation. The integration of deep learning models, adaptive optics, SOCT, and robotic systems could further enhance diagnostic accuracy and patient care in uveitis management. AI-assisted grading systems may improve consistency in AC inflammation scoring and allow remote or technician-led evaluations, although they still require robust clinical validation and regulatory approval. However, it is important to emphasize that the effectiveness of AI depends critically on the quality of input data, the robustness of algorithms, and the rigorous validation of models in diverse clinical settings. Without appropriate training data, standardized imaging protocols, and well-calibrated algorithms, AI tools may yield inaccurate or misleading results.

- *AI-driven automation*:

    - *Artifact suppression*: Deep learning models have been developed to correct various artifacts in OCT imaging, including shadowing, mirror artifacts, saturation, and sunray artifacts [100]. These models can enhance image quality by removing or reducing artifacts that obscure critical details, thereby improving diagnostic accuracy. For example, enhanced super-resolution generative adversarial networks (ESRGAN) have shown promise in correcting saturation artifacts by learning from clear-saturated image pairs, demonstrating robustness and generalization across different tissue types [100].

    - *Cell differentiation*: Radiomics involves extracting quantitative features from OCT images to classify hyperreflective particles in the AC as inflammatory cells, pigments, or debris. This approach leverages machine learning algorithms to analyze texture, intensity, and shape features, potentially overcoming AS-OCT's limitation in differentiating cell types. Combining radiomics with SOCT could further enhance differentiation capabilities by incorporating molecular-level information [38, 101, 102].

- *Advanced imaging technologies*:

    - *Adaptive optics (AO)*: AO-OCT systems offer ultrahigh resolution ($3 \times 3 \times 3\ \mu m^3$) and speed, enabling cellular-level imaging of retinal structures.

While primarily applied to retinal imaging, AO could theoretically be adapted for anterior segment imaging to track inflammatory cell trafficking and trabecular scarring with unprecedented detail, providing insights into uveitis pathophysiology [103, 104].

- *Spectroscopic OCT (SOCT)*: This technology provides molecular profiling capabilities, which can be applied to differentiate granulomatous from non-granulomatous KPs, and reflective points based on their molecular composition. SOCT could enhance diagnostic specificity by identifying unique spectral signatures associated with different types of inflammation, aiding in personalized treatment strategies [4, 26, 105].

- While the primary focus of SOCT in uveitis has been on distinguishing inflammatory cell types, its molecular profiling capabilities also hold the potential for detecting malignant cells. In other fields, such as dermatology and oncology, OCT and spectroscopic techniques have been successfully used to differentiate tumor types such as basal cell carcinoma, squamous cell carcinoma, and breast carcinoma from surrounding normal tissue, based on their unique scattering, absorption, and molecular spectral signatures [106]. For instance, Raman spectroscopy, often integrated with OCT, can achieve nearly 100% accuracy in distinguishing cancer cells from normal cells by analyzing their chemical composition [106].

Translating this approach to uveitis, advanced OCT modalities—such as spectroscopic and polarization-sensitive OCT—could potentially distinguish between hyper-reflective anterior chamber components like pigment granules, red or white blood cells, inflammatory debris, and malignant lymphoid cells. For example, melanin-containing pigment (from iris epithelium or pigmented macrophages) exhibits strong backscattering and depolarization signals, while RBCs have distinct hemoglobin-related absorption, and WBCs demonstrate weaker, diffuse scattering. Malignant cells, as seen in masquerade syndromes such as vitreoretinal lymphoma, may exhibit structural uniformity and altered nuclear-cytoplasmic features detectable through these optical profiles. Future adaptation of tissue-specific spectral libraries and AI-based classifiers may allow OCT to noninvasively characterize intraocular cellular populations and improve diagnostic accuracy in challenging uveitis cases. While these applications remain investigational in uveitis, early-stage research and cross-specialty analogs support their potential for future diagnostic use.

However, applying SOCT to detect malignant cells in the anterior segment of the eye is still experimental and requires further research. The integration of SOCT with other advanced analytic techniques such as radiomics, could potentially enhance its ability to classify various cell types, including malignant ones, by combining molecular information with detailed texture and intensity features extracted from OCT images.

- *Robotic, virtual reality headsets, and contact lens systems*:

  - *Robotic AS-OCT*: Robotic systems can automate AS-OCT imaging, ensuring consistent and artifact-free acquisition even in uncooperative patients. This automation is particularly beneficial in pediatric cases or when rapid imaging is required, as it minimizes the need for manual adjustments and reduces imaging time [9, 107, 108].

- *Portable multifunctional virtual reality headsets in ophthalmic imaging*: Portable multifunctional VR glasses offer a promising solution for ophthalmic imaging, particularly in patients with disabilities or pediatric cases where traditional table-mounted OCT devices are impractical. These systems integrate OCT technology with VR capabilities, providing a comfortable and distraction-free environment for imaging. While not yet commercially available, patented devices like those using superluminescent light-emitting diodes (SLDs) as light sources show potential for enhancing diagnostic accuracy and patient compliance [109]. In pediatric ophthalmology, VR technology is increasingly used to improve diagnosis and treatment experiences by reducing anxiety and enhancing engagement during examinations. Further research is needed to fully integrate these technologies into clinical practice, but they hold significant promise for improving accessibility and reducing costs in ophthalmic care [110–113]. Wearable or miniaturized AS-OCT devices, paired with cloud-based AI analysis, could support longitudinal inflammation tracking and remote monitoring, transforming care for chronic uveitis patients.

- *Gonioscopic or three-mirror contact lens-assisted AS-OCT*: Gonioscopic or three-mirror contact lens-assisted anterior AS-OCT enhances real-time imaging of the ACA, trabecular meshwork, and Schlemm's canal, providing superior visualization compared to standard AS-OCT alone. This approach circumvents limitations such as total internal reflection and improves the resolution of peripheral structures, enabling precise assessment of angle closure, PAS, and TM involvement in conditions like glaucoma and uveitis. The use of contact lenses allows dynamic imaging under physiological conditions, offering valuable insights into aqueous outflow pathways and structural changes. Additionally, this technique holds potential for middle-segment imaging, including the ciliary body and pars plana, which are critical in managing uveitis and other anterior segment pathologies. Middle-segment OCT systems, designed to image the PC, CB, and zonules, may fill the current gap between anterior and posterior segment imaging, particularly in pars planitis or ciliary body granulomas. By combining gonioscopy's broad visualization with AS-OCT's objective and quantitative capabilities, this method represents a significant advancement in anterior segment imaging for both diagnostic and therapeutic applications [114].

- *Standardization initiatives*:

  - *Pediatric normative data*: Establish age-specific reference databases to reduce false positives (e.g., 76% of healthy children show hyperreflective spots) [93]. See Section 6 on Standardization.

  - *Quantitative biomarkers*: Develop metrics like KP volumetry, TM height, and iris smoothness indices for staging and differentiating uveitis subtypes [115, 116].

- *Multimodal integration*:

  - Combine AS-OCT with LFP, UBM, and confocal microscopy for comprehensive diagnostics [117].

By developing multimodal imaging devices combining AS-OCT with AI-driven segmentation, hyperspectral analysis, LFP, Raman spectroscopy, and motion analysis, it will be possible to accurately differentiate inflammatory cells from pigment or debris, enhancing the reliability of AS-OCT in uveitis monitoring and treatment response assessment. Future research should incorporate larger multi-center trials, AI-driven algorithms, and comparative imaging techniques to refine automated AS-OCT's role in routine uveitis management.

Table 4 summarizes key diagnostic AS-OCT findings and their differential implications across uveitis and masquerade syndromes.

7. Conclusions

AS-OCT has rapidly become a transformative tool in the diagnosis and management of uveitis. By offering high-resolution, non-invasive visualization of anterior segment structures, it allows clinicians to detect and quantify features that were once difficult to objectively assess, such as KP morphology, anterior chamber inflammation, and iris changes. These capabilities have already reshaped how we evaluate disease activity and response to treatment in everyday practice.

AS-OCT is not without its challenges. Differences between devices, the absence of cytological and histological validation, limited sensitivity to flare, and difficulties in imaging the CB and PC all highlight the gaps that remain. The inability to consistently differentiate inflammatory cells from debris or pigment, and its sensitivity to motion or mirror artifacts, further complicate its interpretation. These issues reflect the real-world complexity of implementing AS-OCT in diverse clinical settings.

The future of AS-OCT is promising. Integration of SOCT could open doors to molecular-level insights, while adaptive optics may bring us closer to cellular-resolution imaging. AI has the potential to reduce artifacts, standardize segmentation, and make assessments more consistent across users. Perhaps most imaginatively, combining VR technology with OCT, such as through portable multifunctional VR headsets, could offer a distraction-free experience that makes imaging easier in pediatric or uncooperative patients. While still early in development, such systems point to a more accessible and patient-friendly future. Innovations like gonioscopic or three-mirror contact lens-assisted AS-OCT also offer new possibilities for improving middle-segment imaging.

To truly realize this potential, we will need to fill some important gaps like developing normative pediatric datasets, validating new biomarkers such as KP volumetry and iris smoothness indices, and harmonizing protocols across platforms. AS-OCT, even in its current commercially available forms, plays a central role in multimodal assessment of uveitis. It enables detailed evaluation of the cornea, KPs, anterior chamber cells, and angle anatomy—including detection of trabeculitis and ocular hypertension related to corticosteroid use. It also supports iris morphology analysis, helping to differentiate between conditions such as PSS and FUS, and serves as a valuable tool in both pre- and post-cataract evaluation for complex uveitic cases. Color-coded iris cross-sectional imaging may further improve our understanding of inflammatory pathophysiology. Complementary tools such as LFP enhance flare detection and quantification, UBM facilitates visualization of the PC, sulcus, and pars plana, and OCT extends imaging capabilities to the macula, retina, and choroid. Investigational technologies, including confocal microscopy and AO-OCT, offer unique insights at the cellular level. As radiomics and AI-driven analytics become increasingly integrated, we move closer to a fully automated and personalized approach to uveitis care. By addressing current limitations and embracing these emerging innovations, AS-OCT stands to become a cornerstone of precision medicine in uveitis, redefining how we diagnose, monitor, and manage this complex disease spectrum.

Acknowledgements

The authors wish to acknowledge the valuable contributions of Grok 3, ChatGPT v4.0, and Perplexity AI for language polishing. Their advanced language processing tools significantly enhanced the clarity and precision of the manuscript, facilitating the effective communication of our research findings.

Conflict of interest

The authors declare no conflict of interest.

Author details

Joobin Khadamy
Department of Ophthalmology, University Hospital of Umea, Umea, Sweden

*Address all correspondence to: joobin.khadamy@regionvasterbotten.se

References

[1] Regatieri CV, Alwassia A, Zhang JY, et al. Use of optical coherence tomography in the diagnosis and management of uveitis. International Ophthalmology Clinics. 2012;**52**:33-43

[2] Jiao H, Hill LJ, Downie LE, et al. Anterior segment optical coherence tomography: Its application in clinical practice and experimental models of disease. Clinical and Experimental Optometry. 2019;**102**:208-217

[3] Iovino C, Peiretti E, Braghiroli M, et al. Imaging of iris vasculature: Current limitations and future perspective. Eye. 2022;**36**:930-940

[4] Robles FE, Wilson C, Grant G, et al. Molecular imaging true-colour spectroscopic optical coherence tomography. Nature Photonics. 2011;**5**:744-747

[5] Li X, Huang Y, Hao Q. Automated robot-assisted wide-field optical coherence tomography using structured light camera. Biomedical Optics Express. 2023;**14**:4310-4325

[6] Murugan SRB, Sanjay S, Somanath A, et al. Artificial intelligence in uveitis: Innovations in diagnosis and therapeutic strategies. Clinical Ophthalmology. 2024;**18**:3753-3766

[7] Pujari A, Agarwal D, Sharma N. Clinical role of swept source optical coherence tomography in anterior segment diseases: A review. Seminars in Ophthalmology. 2021;**36**:684-691

[8] Mirzayev I, Gündüz AK, Aydın Ellialtıoğlu P, et al. Clinical applications of anterior segment swept-source optical coherence tomography: A systematic review. Photodiagnosis and Photodynamic Therapy. 2023;**42**:103334

[9] Ortiz P, Draelos M, Viehland C, et al. Robotically aligned optical coherence tomography with 5 degree of freedom eye tracking for subject motion and gaze compensation. Biomedical Optics Express. 2021;**12**:7361-7376

[10] Onal S, Tugal-Tutkun I, Neri P, et al. Optical coherence tomography imaging in uveitis. International Ophthalmology. 2014;**34**:401-435

[11] Invernizzi A, Marchi S, Aldigeri R, et al. Objective quantification of anterior chamber inflammation: Measuring cells and flare by anterior segment optical coherence tomography. Ophthalmology. 2017;**124**:1670-1677

[12] Qian Y, Liu L, Shi Y, et al. Assessment of anterior chamber by ultrasound biomicroscopy and anterior segment optical coherence tomography in patients with inflammatory glaucoma. The Journal of International Medical Research. 2019;**47**:5950-5956

[13] Agarwal A, Pichi F, Invernizzi A, et al. Stepwise approach for fundus imaging in the diagnosis and management of posterior uveitis. Survey of Ophthalmology. 2023;**68**:446-480

[14] Ho J, Castro DPE, Castro LC, et al. Clinical assessment of mirror artifacts in spectral-domain optical coherence tomography. Investigative Ophthalmology and Visual Science. 2010;**51**:3714-3720

[15] Steukers L, Glorieux S, Vandekerckhove AP, et al. Diverse microbial interactions with the basement membrane barrier. Trends in Microbiology. 2012;**20**:147-155

[16] Le PM, Mattapallil MJ, Caspi RR, et al. Immunoregulatory properties

of immune cells that associate with the lens capsule surface during acute and resolution phases of experimental autoimmune uveitis. The American Journal of Pathology. 2024;**194**:2194-2211

[17] Khadamy J. Basement membrane alterations in diabetic retinopathy. In: Diabetic Retinopathy - Advancement in Understanding the Pathophysiology and Management Strategies. London, UK: IntechOpen; 2024. Epub ahead of print 17 October 2024. DOI: 10.5772/intechopen.1004632.

[18] Khadamy J. Anterior-segment optical coherence tomography unlocks novel perspectives: Lacking iris anterior limiting layer signal in uveitis. Cureus. 2024;**16**:e51872

[19] Lakshmipathy B, Biswas J. Multimodal imaging of granulomatous anterior uveitis with Berlin nodules due to sarcoidosis. Indian Journal of Ophthalmology Case Reports. 2024;**4**:279-281

[20] Khadamy J. Harnessing the underutilized potential of the lens capsule transplantation in ophthalmology: A narrative review of current applications and future directions. Cureus. 2025;**17**(4):e82259. DOI: 10.7759/cureus.82259

[21] Walker JL, Menko AS. Immune cells in lens injury repair and fibrosis. Experimental Eye Research. 2021;**209**:108664

[22] Herszényi L, Hritz I, Lakatos G, et al. The behavior of matrix metalloproteinases and their inhibitors in colorectal cancer. International Journal of Molecular Sciences. 2012;**13**:13240-13263

[23] Pichi F, Ometto G, Invernizzi A, et al. Automated quantification of uveitic keratic precipitates by use of anterior segment optical coherence tomography. Clinical and Experimental Ophthalmology. 2023;**51**:790-798

[24] Agrawal RV, Murthy S, Sangwan V, et al. Current approach in diagnosis and management of anterior uveitis. Indian Journal of Ophthalmology. 2010;**58**:11-19

[25] Foti R, Zeppieri M, Foti R, et al. Advanced UltraTech approach for distinguishing granulomatous from non-granulomatous corneal endothelial exudates in autoimmune rheumatic anterior uveitis. Journal of Biological Methods. 2024;**11**:e99010034

[26] Hashida N, Asao K, Maruyama K, et al. Cornea findings of spectral domain anterior segment optical coherence tomography in uveitic eyes of various etiologies. Cornea. 2019;**38**:1299-1304

[27] Venkateswaran N, Galor A, Wang J, et al. Optical coherence tomography for ocular surface and corneal diseases: A review. Eye Vision (London). 2018;**5**:13

[28] Kobayashi A, Yokogawa H, Sugiyama K. Optical coherence tomography of band keratopathy. BMJ Case Reports. 2016. **2016**:bcr2016218216. DOI: 10.1136/bcr-2016-218216

[29] Sharma S, Lowder CY, Vasanji A, et al. Automated analysis of anterior chamber inflammation by spectral-domain optical coherence tomography. Ophthalmology. 2015;**122**:1464-1470

[30] Jabs DA, Nussenblatt RB, Rosenbaum JT, et al. Standardization of uveitis nomenclature for reporting clinical data. Results of the first international workshop. American Journal of Ophthalmology. 2005;**140**:509-516

[31] Pillar S, Kadomoto S, Chen K, et al. Automated quantification of anterior

chamber cells using swept-source anterior segment optical coherence tomography. The Journal of Ophthalmic Inflammation and Infection. 2025;**15**:3

[32] Keino H, Aman T, Furuya R, et al. Automated quantitative analysis of anterior segment inflammation using swept-source anterior segment optical coherence tomography: A pilot study. Diagnostics (Basel). 2022;**12**:2703

[33] Baghdasaryan E, Tepelus TC, Marion KM, et al. Analysis of ocular inflammation in anterior chamber-involving uveitis using swept-source anterior segment OCT. International Ophthalmology. 2019;**39**:1793-1801

[34] Li M, Wang H, Liu Y, et al. Comparison of time-domain, spectral-domain and swept-source OCT in evaluating aqueous cells in vitro. Science China. Life Sciences. 2016;**59**:1319-1323

[35] Lu M, Wang X, Lei L, et al. Quantitative analysis of anterior chamber inflammation using the novel CASIA2 optical coherence tomography. American Journal of Ophthalmology. 2020;**216**:59-68

[36] Igbre AO, Rico MC, Garg SJ. High-speed optical coherence tomography as a reliable adjuvant tool to grade ocular anterior chamber inflammation. Retina. 2014;**34**:504-508

[37] Sorkhabi MA, Potapenko IO, Ilginis T, et al. Assessment of anterior uveitis through anterior-segment optical coherence tomography and artificial intelligence-based image analyses. Translational Vision Science and Technology. 2022;**11**:7

[38] Bellchambers A, Shu R, Chu CJ, et al. Differentiation of anterior chamber pigment and inflammatory cells using swept-source optical coherence tomography: A cross-sectional study. Eye. 2025. Epub ahead of print 12 March 2025. DOI: 10.1038/s41433-025-03697-2

[39] Rose-Nussbaumer J, Li Y, Lin P, et al. Aqueous cell differentiation in anterior uveitis using Fourier-domain optical coherence tomography. Investigative Ophthalmology and Visual Science. 2015;**56**:1430-1436

[40] Mahendradas P, Chauhan S, Kawali A, et al. Iris crystals: A rare clinical finding in chronic anterior uveitis. Middle East African Journal of Ophthalmology. 2019;**26**:46-48

[41] Escribano López P, González Guijarro JJ. Comparative analysis of iridian anterior segment OCT and microbiological features in Fuchs uveitis syndrome and Posner-Schlossman syndrome. Arbeitsphysiologie [Internet]. 7 Jan 2025. Epub ahead of print. DOI: 10.1007/s00417-024-06714-4

[42] Cai Y, Wu W, Wang Y, et al. Anterior segment structures in dark iris Chinese patients with unilateral Fuchs' uveitis syndrome. International Ophthalmology. 2022;**42**:2939-2947

[43] Callear AB, Reynolds A, Harry J, et al. Iris crystals in chronic uveitis. The British Journal of Ophthalmology. 1999;**83**:703-706

[44] Cho WJ, Kim Y, Kim JD, et al. Association of trabecular meshwork height with steroid-induced ocular hypertension. Scientific Reports. 2023;**13**:9143

[45] Cho WJ, Shin HJ, Kim M, et al. Clinical prediction nomogram for steroid-induced ocular hypertension risk in patients with intravitreal dexamethasone implant. Heliyon. 2024;**10**:e34635

[46] Soliman W, Nassr MA, Abdelazeem K, et al. Appearance of herpes simplex keratitis on anterior segment optical coherence tomography. International Ophthalmology. 2019;**39**:2923-2928

[47] Karmiris E, Papakonstantinou E, Tsiripidis K, et al. Atypical phacolytic glaucoma diagnosed by biometry and anterior segment optical coherence tomography (OCT) in a patient with CMV anterior uveitis. European Journal of Ophthalmology. 2024;**34**:NP29–NP32

[48] Yan X, Li M, Wang J, et al. Morphology of the trabecular meshwork and Schlemm's canal in Posner-Schlossman syndrome. Investigative Ophthalmology and Visual Science. 2022;**63**:1

[49] Lippera M, Nicolosi C, Vannozzi L, et al. The role of anterior segment optical coherence tomography in uveitis-glaucoma-hyphema syndrome. European Journal of Ophthalmology. 2022;**32**:2211-2218

[50] Hashida N, Terubayashi A, Ohguro N. Anterior segment optical coherence tomography findings of presumed intraocular tuberculosis. Cutaneous and Ocular Toxicology. 2011;**30**:75-77

[51] Alsobaie NA, Almohizea AI, Al-Zahrani Y, et al. Goniosynechialysis for secondary angle closure glaucoma in aphakic patient after pars plana vitrectomy. The American Journal of Ophthalmology Case Reports. 2018;**12**:15-17

[52] Lutsenko N, Isakova O, Rudycheva O, et al. Preoperative OCT lens evaluation in posterior subcapsular cataract - prevention of complications from phacoemulsification. Arbeitsphysiologie. 2025;**263**:443-450

[53] Wang X, Dong J, Zhang S, et al. OCT application before and after cataract surgery. In: OCT - Applications in Ophthalmology. London, UK: IntechOpen; 2018. Epub ahead of print 19 September 2018. DOI: 10.5772/intechopen.77281.

[54] Al-Essa RS, Alfawaz AM. New insights into cataract surgery in patients with uveitis: A detailed review of the current literature. Saudi Journal of Ophthalmology. 2022;**36**:133-141

[55] Macovei ML, Canache M, Neagoe B-M. Phacolytic glaucoma - Case report. Romanian Journal of Ophthalmology. 2021;**65**:191-195

[56] Werner L, Michelson J, Ollerton A, et al. Anterior segment optical coherence tomography in the assessment of postoperative intraocular lens optic changes. Journal of Cataract and Refractive Surgery. 2012;**38**:1077-1085

[57] Muñoz-Solano J, Tondini G, Zicarelli F, et al. Utility of anterior segment OCT in the management of uveitic cataract surgery: A fibrinoid syndrome case treated with rtPA. Ocular Immunology and Inflammation. 2024;**32**:1128-1131

[58] Payá EM, González MA, Ortuño MR, et al. AS-OCT of cyclitic membrane pre and post treatment with rtPA in the anterior chamber. Romanian Journal of Ophthalmology. 2022;**66**:191-192

[59] Grzybowski A, Markeviciute A, Zemaitiene R. A narrative review of intraocular lens opacifications: Update 2020. The Annals of Translational Medicine. 2020;**8**:1547

[60] Invernizzi A, Zaffalon C, Manni P, Zicarelli F, Chisari D, Adani C, et al. Anterior vitreous objective assessment in uveitis: An anterior segment swept

source optical coherence tomography study. Ocular Immunology and Inflammation [Internet]. 2025;**33**(1):24-32. DOI: 10.1080/09273948.2024.2339435

[61] Gozzi F, Bertolini M, Gentile P, et al. Artificial intelligence-assisted processing of anterior segment OCT images in the diagnosis of vitreoretinal lymphoma. Diagnostics (Basel); 2023;**13**(14):2451. Epub ahead of print 23 July 2023. DOI: 10.3390/diagnostics13142451

[62] Mahendradas P, Avadhani K, Ramachandran S, et al. Anterior segment optical coherence tomography findings of iris granulomas in Hansen's disease: A case report. The Journal of Ophthalmic Inflammation and Infection. 2013;**3**:36

[63] Li Y, Tan O, Brass R, et al. Corneal epithelial thickness mapping by Fourier-domain optical coherence tomography in normal and keratoconic eyes. Ophthalmology. 2012;**119**:2425-2433

[64] Yu S, You D, Agrawal R, et al. Noninvasive diagnosis of viral keratouveitis with retro-corneal endothelial plaques: A case series. Ocular Immunology and Inflammation. 2022;**30**:1482-1488

[65] Arora T, Sharma N, Arora S, et al. Fulminant herpetic keratouveitis with flap necrosis following laser in situ keratomileusis: Case report and review of literature. Journal of Cataract and Refractive Surgery. 2014;**40**:2152-2156

[66] Avila MY, Gallego-Suarez LJ. Confocal microscopy, anterior segment optical coherence tomography and clinical findings in a non-granulomatous uveitis case for mpox infection. Ocular Immunology and Inflammation. 2024;**32**:1901-1903

[67] Escribano Lopez P, Gonzalez Guijarro JJ. Iridian anterior segment OCT in rubella uveitis syndrome and cytomegalovirus anterior uveitis: A comparative study. Arbeitsphysiologie. 2022;**260**:3647-3655

[68] Chen JL, Tessema R, Emami-Naeini P, et al. A vascular syphilitic iris lesion. The American Journal of Ophthalmology Case Reports. 2023;**31**:101858

[69] Rosenberg CR, Pasadhika S. A vascularized iris mass in ocular syphilis: A case report and review of literature. Ocular Immunology and Inflammation. 2024;**32**:1648-1654

[70] Knape RM, Sayyad FE, Davis JL. Moxifloxacin and bilateral acute iris transillumination. The Journal of Ophthalmic Inflammation and Infection. 2013;**3**:10

[71] Davis JL, Taskintuna I, Freeman WR, et al. Iritis and hypotony after treatment with intravenous cidofovir for cytomegalovirus retinitis. Archives of Ophthalmology. 1997;**115**:733-737

[72] Galvis V, Shields TA, et al. Spontaneous regression of a primary iris stromal cyst in a patient with keratoconus. A case report. Ceská a Slovenská Oftalmologie. 2021;**77**:253-256

[73] Kitazawa K, Nagata K, Yamanaka Y, et al. Diffuse anterior retinoblastoma with sarcoidosis-like nodule. Case Reports Ophthalmology. 2015;**6**:443-447

[74] Shao YF, Echegaray JJ, Singh AD. Metastatic tumors of the uvea. In: Intraocular Tumors. Singapore: Springer Singapore; 2024. pp. 179-185

[75] Ferry AP, Font RL. Carcinoma metastatic to the eye and orbit. I. A clinicopathologic study of 227 cases. Archives of Ophthalmology. 1974;**92**:276-286

[76] Mitamura M, Kase S, Suimon Y, et al. A case of metastatic iris tumor observed

with anterior segment optical coherence tomography before and after radiation therapy. In Vivo. 2020;**34**:2159-2162

[77] Gündüz AK, Mirzayev I, Okcu Heper A, et al. Anterior segment optical coherence tomography in ocular surface tumours and simulating lesions. Eye. 2023;**37**:925-937

[78] Akbaş E, Barut Selver Ö, Palamar M. Retrospective evaluation of corneal foreign bodies with anterior segment optical coherence tomography. Turkish Journal of Ophthalmology. 2021;**51**:265-268

[79] Mahmoud A, Messaoud R, Abid F, et al. Anterior segment optical coherence tomography and retained vegetal intraocular foreign body masquerading as chronic anterior uveitis. The Journal of Ophthalmic Inflammation and Infection. 2017;**7**:13

[80] Celebi ARC, Kilavuzoglu AE, Altiparmak UE, et al. The role of anterior segment optical coherence tomography in the management of an intra-corneal foreign body. Springerplus. 2016;**5**:1559

[81] Agarwal R, Rana N, Beri S, et al. Insect wing case corneal foreign body: ASOCT-based findings. BML Case Reports. 2022;**15**:e251578

[82] Kitahata M, Suzuki T, Oka N, et al. Anterior segment optical coherence tomography of patients with late-onset tunnel fungal infections with endophthalmitis after cataract surgery. Cornea. 2016;**35**:1138-1140

[83] Durkin SR, Chappell A, Craig JE. Anterior segment optical coherence tomography in the investigation of an unusual case of entoptic phenomenon. Clinical and Experimental Ophthalmology. 2008;**36**:796-797

[84] Cauduro RS, C do A F, MSÁ M, et al. Application of anterior segment optical coherence tomography in pediatric ophthalmology. Journal of Ophthalmology. 2012;**2012**:313120

[85] Akbarali S, Rahi JS, Dick AD, et al. Imaging-based uveitis surveillance in juvenile idiopathic arthritis: Feasibility, acceptability, and diagnostic performance. Arthritis and Rhematology. 2021;**73**:330-335

[86] Diala FGI, McCarthy K, Chen JL, et al. Multimodal imaging in pediatric uveitis. Therapeutic Advances in Ophthalmology. 2021;**13**:25158414211059244

[87] Soliman W, Wasfi EI, Ali OM. Spectral domain optical coherence tomography study of pearl-like lesions in the anterior chamber. Clinical Ophthalmology. 2012;**6**:903-907

[88] Dave S, Rahi JS, Petrushkin H, et al. UVESCREEN1: A randomised feasibility study of imaging-based uveitis screening for children with juvenile idiopathic arthritis- study protocol. PLoS One. 2025;**20**:e0316410

[89] Tsui E, Chen JL, Jackson NJ, et al. Quantification of anterior chamber cells in children with uveitis using anterior segment optical coherence tomography. American Journal of Ophthalmology. 2022;**241**:254-261

[90] Etherton K, Rahi JS, Petrushkin H, et al. Quantitative and qualitative assessment of anterior segment optical coherence tomography capture of disease state in childhood anterior uveitis. The British Journal of Ophthalmology. 2023;**107**:966-972

[91] Uthayananthan P, Tanwar N, Rahi JS, et al. Imaging-based detection of anterior chamber inflammation: A

comparative diagnostic accuracy study. American Journal of Ophthalmology. 2025;**270**:131-139

[92] Concilio M, Cennamo G, Giordano M, et al. Anterior segment-optical coherence tomography features in Blau syndrome. Photodiagnosis and Photodynamic Therapy. 2021;**34**:102278

[93] Solebo AL, Bellchambers A, Kellett S, et al. Establishing the normative data set necessary for imaging-based childhood uveitis surveillance: A cross-sectional study. Investigative Ophthalmology and Visual Science. 2024;**65**:9

[94] Maring M, Saraf SS, Blazes M, et al. Grading anterior chamber inflammation with anterior segment optical coherence tomography: An overview. Ocular Immunology and Inflammation. 2022;**30**:357-363

[95] Santos-Oliveira J, Teixeira-Martins R, Ferreira AM, et al. Anterior segment optical coherence tomography evaluation of a dexamethasone intravitreal implant in the crystalline lens: A case report. The International Medical Case Reports Journal. 2025;**18**:27-32

[96] Kelgaonkar A, Pathengay A, Patel A. Anterior segment OCT (AS-OCT) imaging characteristics in cases of uveitis. Indian Journal of Ophthalmology - Case Reports. 2024;**4**:584-584

[97] Solebo AL, Barry RJ, Keane PA, et al. Under-utilisation of reproducible, child appropriate or patient reported outcome measures in childhood uveitis interventional research. Orphanet Journal of Rare Diseases. 2019;**14**:125

[98] Torm MEW, Sander B, Hornum M, et al. Characterization of hyperreflective dots by structural and angiographic optical coherence tomography in patients with diabetic retinopathy and healthy subjects. Journal of Clinical Medicine. 2022;**11**:6646

[99] Chen L, Cao D, Messinger JD, et al. Histology and clinical imaging lifecycle of black pigment in fibrosis secondary to neovascular age-related macular degeneration. Experimental Eye Research. 2022;**214**:108882

[100] Hu M, Yuan Z, Yang D, et al. Deep learning-based inpainting of saturation artifacts in optical coherence tomography images. Journal of Innovative Optical Health Sciences. 2024;**17**(3):2350026. DOI: 10.1142/s1793545823500268

[101] Hu Y, Meng Y, Liang Y, et al. Machine learning and optical-coherence-tomography-derived radiomics analysis to predict the postoperative anatomical outcome of full-thickness macular hole. Bioengineering (Basel). 2024;**11**:949

[102] Sil Kar S, Cetin H, Srivastava SK, et al. Optical coherence tomography-derived texture-based radiomics features identify eyes with intraocular inflammation in the HAWK clinical trial. Heliyon. 2024;**10**:e32232

[103] Liu Y, Crowell JA, Kurokawa K, et al. Ultrafast adaptive optics for imaging the living human eye. Nature Communications. 2024;**15**:10409

[104] Miller DT, Kocaoglu OP, Wang Q, et al. Adaptive optics and the eye (super resolution OCT). Eye. 2011;**25**:321-330

[105] Widaatalla Y, Wolswijk T, Khan MD, et al. Radiomics in dermatological optical coherence tomography (OCT): Feature repeatability, reproducibility, and integration into diagnostic models in a prospective study. Cancers (Basel). 2025;**17**(5):768. Epub ahead of print 24 February 2025. DOI: 10.3390/cancers17050768

[106] You C, Yi J-Y, Hsu T-W, et al. Integration of cellular-resolution optical coherence tomography and Raman spectroscopy for discrimination of skin cancer cells with machine learning. Journal of Biomedical Optics. 2023;**28**:096005

[107] Song A, Roh K-M, Lusk JB, et al. Robotic optical coherence tomography retinal imaging for emergency department patients: A pilot study for emergency physicians' diagnostic performance. Annals of Emergency Medicine. 2023;**81**:501-508

[108] Fang R, Zhang P, Zhang T, et al. Freeform robotic optical coherence tomography beyond the optical field-of-view limit. bioRxivorg. 2024;**2024.2005.2021**:595073. Epub ahead of print 23 May 2024. DOI: 10.1101/2024.05.21.595073

[109] Liu J. A multifunctional VR glasses for portable ophthalmic OCT medical diagnosis. CN:110742575:B. 2022. Available from: https://patents.google.com/patent/CN110742575B/en [Accessed: March 23, 2025]

[110] Nikolaidou A, Sandali A, Chatzidimitriou E, et al. Virtual reality with eye tracking for pediatric ophthalmology: A systematic review. Journal of Pediatric Ophthalmology and Strabismus. 2024;**61**:381-390

[111] Foust J, McCloud M, Narawane A, et al. New directions for ophthalmic OCT - Handhelds, surgery, and robotics. Translational Vision Science and Technology. 2025;**14**:14

[112] Bozchalooi IS, Emami-Naeini P. Head-Mounted Device Including Display for Fully-Automated Ophthalmic Imaging. 2022. p. 217160. Available from: https://patentscope.wipo.int/search/en/detail.jsf?docId=WO2022217160 [Accessed: March 23, 2025]

[113] Maloca PM, Williams EA, Mushtaq F, et al. Feasibility and tolerability of ophthalmic virtual reality as a medical communication tool in children and young people. Acta Ophthalmologica. 2022;**100**:e588-e597

[114] Keller MJ, Gast TJ, King BJ. Advancements in high-resolution imaging of the iridocorneal angle. Frontiers in Ophthalmology (Lausanne). 2023;**3**:1229670

[115] Kanavi MR, Soheilian M. Confocal scan features of keratic precipitates in granulomatous versus nongranulomatous uveitis. Journal of Ophthalmic and Vision Research. 2011;**6**:255-258

[116] Zarei M, Pour EK, Ebrahimiadib N, Riazi-Esfahani H. Quantitative analysis of the iris surface smoothness by spectral domain optical coherence tomography in Fuchs uveitis. medRxiv; 2020. DOI: 10.1101/2020.05.06.20093302. Preprint of: Ocular immunology and inflammation. 2022;**30**(3):697-702

[117] Siak J, Mahendradas P, Chee S-P. Multimodal imaging in anterior uveitis. Ocular Immunology and Inflammation. 2017;**25**:434-446

Section 2

Disease-Specific Reviews

Chapter 3

Tuberculous Uveitis: An Overview of Diagnosis and Management

Roha Ahmad Choudhary

Abstract

Tuberculous uveitis (TBU) is an important cause of infectious uveitis, particularly in TB-endemic regions, such as South Asia, which have a significant and heavy burden of disease. It results from hematogenous spread of *Mycobacterium tuberculosis* (MTB) to the uveal tract and presents with a broad spectrum of clinical phenotypes. Due to its paucibacillary nature and varied presentations, TBU poses significant diagnostic challenges, often leading to delayed treatment and increased risk of visual impairment. This chapter will offer an overview of TBU, highlighting key diagnostic tools and evidence-based treatment approaches, which will help guide clinicians in timely recognition and management, improving patient outcomes through early diagnosis and appropriate intervention.

Keywords: tuberculosis, TB uveitis, TB uveitis-imaging and diagnosis, TB uveitis-management, TB uveitis-prevalence

1. Introduction

Tuberculosis (TB) is one of the most prevalent infectious diseases around the world and has an especially high burden of disease in developing countries [1]. Infection of the eye and the adnexa by the *M. tuberculosis* is classified as ocular TB and specific involvement of the uveal layer is one of its manifestations. TB uveitis (TBU) usually occurs because of spread of bacteria through blood to the vascular uveal layer rather than as a primary infection [2, 3]. Globally, it is estimated that around one-quarter of the population has been infected with either active or latent TB [4]. According to World Health Organization (WHO) Global tuberculosis report 2024, TB was the most lethal infectious organism reported across the globe and a leading cause of morbidity and mortality. Majority of the TB infections affect the lungs, but it can also cause disease in other organs including the eye. In 2019, around 16% of the total new TB infections reported were extrapulmonary [5, 6]. TB is a known cause of infectious uveitis, particularly in countries of high disease burden. According to estimates, ocular TB prevalence in patients with pulmonary TB is around 1%, whereas in extrapulmonary TB the percentage increases to around 20% [7]. TB uveitis is different from other types of TB because of the paucibacillary nature of the organism when it affects the eye and the diverse clinical presentations [8]. It can affect different segments of the eye and have various presentations, such as anterior, intermediate, panuveitis, retinal vasculitis, choroidal lesions, serpiginous-like choroiditis (SLC), among others. Diagnostic challenges associated with TB uveitis can lead to a delay in treatment, which may cause poorer outcomes and long-term visual damage. In this chapter, we discuss the epidemiology, clinical manifestations, diagnostic approach (including new advances), and management—from standard therapy to novel local treatments—of TB uveitis.

A detailed literature search using the PubMed database over the last 10 years was performed. The following keywords were used to perform the search: "TB uveitis," "tuberculous uveitis," "TB uveitis management," "TB uveitis treatment," "anterior TB uveitis," "intermediate TB uveitis," "posterior TB uveitis," "TB retinal vasculitis," "TB panuveitis," "serpiginous-like choroiditis," "choroidal tuberculoma," "TB retinal vasculitis," "Eales disease AND TB." These terms were used alone and in various combinations.

2. TB uveitis prevalence

Even though there was a reduction of 9% from 2015 to 2019 in total cases worldwide, TB remains a disease of significance in several low-income countries, such as India, Bangladesh, Pakistan, and Indonesia [5]. TB is often considered as a common cause of infectious uveitis in TB-endemic regions. However, the exact incidence is hard to establish as the data are lacking. Ishaq et al. reported that 48% of total cases of uveitis seen in a tertiary care hospital in Karachi, Pakistan, had infectious etiology and 50.6% of classified cases were due to TB, which far exceeded any other cause [9]. North America is said to have the lowest prevalence of tuberculosis as compared to Europe and Asian countries [10]. Hong et al. published a review of 141 patients, who presented to them with uveitis at University of Southern California in Los Angeles [11]. They reported that only 4.3% of these patients had a diagnosis of ocular TB. It is worth mentioning that this number was significantly higher than what is usually seen in patient population in the United States, data presented by Patel et al. showed that over a period of 15 years only 0.7% of uveitis patients had a presumed diagnosis of TB uveitis [12].

Al-Qarni et al. reported 141 eyes were diagnosed with TBU in their university hospital in Saudi Arabia, during a period of 17 years from 1996 to 2013. Fifty-six percent of the reported patients had panuveitis, with posterior uveitis being the second most common type (24.1%) [13]. As many as 7.1% and 12.8% of the cases had anterior and intermediate uveitis, respectively. They reported a significant delay in diagnosis from the start of symptoms, which highlights the challenges and difficulties associated with diagnosing TB uveitis. On average, patients had symptoms for around 7 months before a diagnosis was reached. They attributed this delay to the reason that it is difficult to isolate and test *M. tuberculosis* and TB uveitis often imitates other conditions in its presentation.

Mao et al. present data from their study in Beijing, China, of patients presenting with chronic posterior uveitis with no definite diagnosis [14]. Their patients who had either a positive tuberculin skin test (TST) or interferon gamma release assay (IGRA) test were given a trial of anti-tuberculous therapy (ATT). Out of 84 patients, 46 were diagnosed with TB uveitis as they responded to the treatment. This number shows the importance of keeping TB uveitis as a differential diagnosis in non-responding or recurrent uveitis cases.

Krassas et al. report data from Manchester, UK, which is a non-TB-endemic area [15]. The results were gathered for a period from 2008 to 2015 and included 48 patients who were confirmed to have TB uveitis. The interesting finding was that 75% of these patients were those who were born outside the UK, with 46% from either India or Pakistan. These data show that majority of the cases found even in non-endemic regions are primarily from the ethnic minorities born in high TB prevalence regions. Therefore, it can be suggested that such patients even when seen in low endemic settings should have work-up and treatment for TB uveitis with a low threshold. British Ophthalmological Surveillance Unit (BOSU) gathered data from hospitals in the UK from October 2016 till November 2017. Similarly, their data set showed that 71% of the patients with TB uveitis were born overseas and the overall incidence of ocular TB was calculated to be 0.73 per million population per annum [16]. Another study from a non-endemic region reported similar findings. Ng et al. reported a case series of patients from New Zealand, 97% of their patients were born outside New Zealand, with 88% of these being Asians [17]. Thirty-three percent of these patients had posterior uveitis and anterior uveitis being second at 26%. The study was based in Auckland, which is the most populous city of New Zealand, and has a TB incident rate of 14.6 per 100,000 as compared to 7 per 100,000 for New Zealand overall [18]. Darian Smith's data from Australia for a period of 10 years (2005–2016) showed a similar demographic distribution. In their case, 96% of the TB uveitis cases were reported in those who were born outside Australia with an incidence of 0.077 per 100,000 per year [19].

In summary, while the exact incidence of ocular TB is hard to ascertain, these studies collectively indicate that TBU is a significant cause of uveitis especially in TB-endemic populations and in immigrants from high-prevalence regions, often with diagnosis delayed due to its protean manifestations.

3. TB uveitis types (classification)

TBU is divided into anterior, intermediate, posterior, and panuveitis according to the Standardization of Uveitis Nomenclature (SUN) Working Group classification [20]. Common clinical features vary with the involved segment and may include granulomatous anterior inflammation with extensive posterior synechiae, intermediate uveitis with vitreous opacities, or posterior segment involvement, such as retinal vasculitis, choroidal tuberculomas, and serpiginous-like choroiditis (see **Table 1**) [21]. In the absence of an internationally accepted gold standard test, each center or clinician relies on their own criteria. Gupta et al. report one such system or hierarchy of diagnostic measures devised in their center. They include four categories of evidence i.e. (A) Clinical signs. (B) Ocular investigations (positive polymerase chain reaction (PCR) or acid-fast bacilli (AFB)/culture of *M. tuberculosis* from the ocular sample). (C) Systemic investigations (positive chest X-ray (CXR), Mantoux test, or evidence of extrapulmonary TB). (D) Therapeutic test (by assessing the response to ATT) [22]. Clinical signs form the basis for initial suspicion of TB infection; however, further evidence was often needed because ATT could be potentially toxic [23].

3.1 Anterior and intermediate tuberculous uveitis

Anterior TB uveitis can manifest either unilaterally or bilaterally with features, such as keratic precipitates, iris nodules, synechiae, and rarely hypopyon [24].

Clinical type	Features	Complications	Recommended treatments
Anterior TB uveitis	Unilateral or bilateral; keratic precipitates; iris nodules (Koeppe and Busacca); synechiae; rarely hypopyon	Chronic disease; recurrent; cataract formation	Anti-tuberculous therapy (ATT); steroids
Intermediate TB uveitis	Vitritis; snowball opacities; vascular sheathing	Cataract formation; vitreous exudates (snow banking)	ATT; steroids
Posterior TB uveitis	Inflammation of the choroid	Retinal detachment, optic nerve damage	ATT; steroids
Panuveitis	Involvement of all uveal tract segments	As above	ATT; steroids
Serpiginous-like choroiditis	Placoid lesions; vitritis; foveal sparing	As above	ATT; steroids; can benefit from local therapy.
Choroidal tuberculoma	Yellow mass under the retina; size 4 to 14 mm	Confused with malignancy, hemangiomas, or metastasis	ATT; steroids
Retinal vasculitis	Inflammation of retinal vasculature; neovascularization; vitreous hemorrhage; fibrous proliferation; tractional retinal detachment	Similar presentation: Eales disease	ATT; steroids; anti-VEGF (in CNV, ischaemic neovascularization, or CME); laser; vitrectomy

Table 1.
Clinical types of TB uveitis.

Anterior TB uveitis usually presents as a chronic disease and is often recurrent. Iris nodules are also a feature; those found on the margins are called Koeppe nodules and those on the surface of the iris are called Busacca nodules [25]. Intermediate uveitis is defined as inflammation of the vitreous, which presents with features like vitritis, snowball opacities, and vascular sheathing, among others. It can be associated with both infectious and non-infectious aetiologies, with TB being the leading infectious cause in endemic regions [6, 26]. Cataract formation is a common complication of intermediate TB uveitis, with Babu et al. reporting a rare complication of vitreous exudates, also known as snow banking [27].

3.2 Posterior uveitis and panuveitis

Posterior segment is most frequently affected by TB uveitis as choroid has a rich oxygen supply, which aids the growth of *M. tuberculosis*. This was supported by Patel et al. in their retrospective case series of 26 eyes, out of which 20 had either posterior or panuveitis over a period of 15 years [12]. An interesting finding with TB posterior uveitis is that inflammation may be a result of immune response rather than direct invasion by the organism and hence ATT alone may not be very effective [24].

3.3 Serpiginous-like choroiditis

Serpiginous-like choroiditis (SLC) involves inflammation of the retinal pigment epithelium and inner choroidal layers as a result of TB infection [28]. It often presents bilaterally with multiple foci, which then take a "serpiginoid" form (as described by

Jain et al.) [29]. Another presentation involves placoid lesions, which spread outward from the center. Presence of vitritis and foveal sparing are common features of SLC and tend to affect young to middle-aged patients [30]. It is believed they occur as a result of immune response to the *M. tuberculosis* rather than direct invasion of the choroidal tissue by the organism [31].

3.4 Choroidal tuberculoma

Choroidal tuberculomas are one of the most common manifestations of ocular TB and have a high incidence, especially with systemic disseminated TB. Histopathologic evaluation of these tuberculomas has revealed the presence of MTB organism in the typical caseating granulomas [25]. Choroidal tuberculomas are often confused with malignancy, hemangiomas, or metastasis but their characteristic fundus appearance aid with the often challenging diagnosis. Tuberculomas appear as a yellow-looking mass under the retina, which may range in size from 4 to 14 mm [32].

3.5 Tubercular retinal vasculitis and Eales disease

Retinal vasculitis involves the inflammation of either arterial or venous vasculature of the retina. Along with infectious causes such as TB, it can be due to non-infectious inflammatory conditions or idiopathic disorder [33]. Retinal vasculitis caused by TB often results in complications, such as neovascularization, vitreous hemorrhage, fibrous proliferation, and tractional retinal detachment. In local data presented by Apinyawasisuk et al. from Thailand, the leading infectious cause behind retinal vasculitis was TB (6/14 patients) and non-infectious cause was Eales disease (23/47) [33]. Eales disease is an idiopathic disorder with ophthalmic features similar to retinal vasculitis caused by the *M. tuberculosis* (e.g., peri-phlebitis). It presents with vasculitis, neovascularization, venous occlusion, and recurrent vitreous hemorrhage [34, 35]. Several studies have shown *Mycobacterium* species to be detected in polymerase chain reactions (PCRs) performed on samples from those diagnosed with Eales disease [36–38]. Singh et al. in India reported that 57.14% of those diagnosed with Eales disease had shown presence of the *M. tuberculosis* organism on vitreous fluid PCR tests [39]. Due to similar presentations of both, Eales disease is treated in a similar fashion to TB retinal vasculitis with steroids, ATT, anti-VEGF (vascular endothelial growth factor), laser, or vitrectomy, depending on the severity at presentation. Many researchers believe Eales disease is a form of TB vasculitis, which is TB negative on traditional testing.

It should be noted that these clinical forms are not pathognomonic for TB; thus, in practice, clinicians must often treat these presentations as presumptive TBU in the appropriate context (as definitive proof of mycobacteria is rarely obtained).

4. TB uveitis diagnostic testing

TBU often evades an absolute diagnosis and hence appropriate treatment, due to difficulties caused by an absence of an easy-to-perform gold standard test. Diagnosing TBU remains the biggest challenge in dealing with the disease and specialists majorly rely on clinical features and classifications. Some clinicians rely on therapeutic response as a measure to confirm the presence of TB; however, this does not answer the need for accurate diagnostics. Often, a decision to initiate therapy is made based on the overall picture, including exposure to TB, past medical history, imaging, and diagnostic test results (see **Table 2**). Definitive diagnosis is performed by ocular tissue sampling, which is an invasive procedure and not without serious risks [2].

There are several commercially available tests for diagnosis of TB infection, among which tuberculin skin test (TST) is the one that has been in use for the longest time. However, it has low specificity, especially in endemic populations, because of BCG (Bacille Calmette-Guérin) vaccinations, high infection rate with non-tuberculous mycobacteria, and low reliability due to inter-reader variability in administration and reporting of the results [40, 41]. Interferon gamma release assays (IGRAs) are newer blood tests that involve testing a sample for the level of Interferon Gamma (IFN-γ) produced by T cells sensitized to specific MTB antigens. Compared to TST, it eliminates errors caused by user bias, need for an additional visit, and therefore has increasingly replaced TST as the test of choice [6, 42]. IGRAs can help differentiate true TB infection from a false-positive TST due to prior BCG vaccination. There are two types of Food and Drug Administration (FDA)-approved IGRA tests available, namely; QuantiFERON TB assay (Cellestis/Qiagen, Carnegie, Australia) and T-SPOT.

Test	Method	Sensitivity/specificity	Clinical utility
Tuberculin skin test (TST)	Injection of tuberculin and measuring the skin reaction	Low specificity in endemic populations due to BCG vaccination and non-tuberculous mycobacteria.	Used for initial screening but has limitations in accuracy
Interferon gamma release assays (IGRAs)	Blood test measuring IFN-γ produced by T cells	QuantiFERON-TB GIT assay: Sensitivity 64%, specificity 99.5%. T-SPOT.TB: sensitivity 67%, specificity 91%.	Preferred over TST for its higher accuracy and ability to differentiate between TB and BCG vaccination
Polymerase chain reaction (PCR)	Detection of MTB DNA in ocular samples	Sensitivity: 88%, specificity: 71%	Useful in challenging diagnostic cases but not recommended for routine use. Performance variability ranging from 37% to 88%.
Chest X-ray (CXR)	Imaging of the chest	Sensitivity: 14.7%, specificity: 94.3%	Routinely used in evaluation but has weak diagnostic accuracy for TB uveitis but good for pulmonary TB.
Optical coherence tomography (OCT)	Imaging of the retina and choroid	Ancillary, not diagnostic test	Provides high-quality cross-sectional images, useful in managing retinal pathologies
OCT angiography (OCT-A)	Combines OCT with angiography	Ancillary, not diagnostic test	Detects blood flow impairment and complications like choroidal neovascularization
Molecular tools	GeneXpert MTB/RIF, GeneXpert ultra assay	GeneXpert ultra is reported to have better performance in detecting ocular TB as compared to GeneXpert MTB/RIF.	Detects MTB using nucleic acid amplification

Table 2.
Diagnostic tools for TB uveitis.

TB assay (Oxford Immunotec, Oxford, UK) [43]. QuantiFERON-TB Gold Plus (QFT-Plus; Qiagen, Hilden, Germany) is a fourth-generation IGRA test, which is based on an enzyme-linked immunosorbent assay (ELISA) for IFN-γ [44, 45]. On the other hand, T-SPOT.TB is based on an enzyme-linked immunospot (ELISpot) assay for detecting cells that produce IFN-γ [46]. Notably, IGRA (and TST) only indicate infection at some point and remain positive, even after successful treatment. Therefore, in TB-endemic regions or previously treated individuals, a positive test must be interpreted with caution and in conjunction with clinical and radiologic findings. A study conducted in Singapore compared the diagnostic accuracy between the two types of IGRAs and concluded QuantiFERON-TB Gold In-Tube (QFT-GIT) (sensitivity 64%, specificity 99.5%) to be more specific but less sensitive than T-SPOT.TB (sensitivity 67%, specificity 91%) [21].

Nora et al. performed a meta-analysis to assess the diagnostic accuracy of PCR for diagnosing TB uveitis. They reported a pooled positivity rate of 0.55 (95% confidence interval (CI) 0.44–0.67), sensitivity of 88% (95% CI 83–92), and specificity of 71% (95% CI 60–80). They concluded the inefficacy of PCR as a routine test for TB uveitis and may only be beneficial in cases with diagnostic challenges [47]. The Collaborative Ocular Tuberculosis Study (COTS-1, Report 3) analyses and discusses the group of patients (59 out of 962 sample population) from their study who underwent PCR of intraocular samples for TB uveitis. Thirty-three out of 59 had a positive PCR result, out of these 22 (n:30) patients had a concurrent positive TST, 4 (n:33) had a positive QFT-Gold test, and one had positive T-Spot.TB test [48]. GeneXpert MTB/RIF (rifampicin), GeneXpert Ultra assay, and *Mycobacterium tuberculosis* drug resistance (MTBDR) plus assay have been used to test for *M. tuberculosis* on ocular samples in some studies [49, 50].

Even those tests that are available are not always accurately indicative of active ocular infection. Nora et al. proposed the use of type 1 IFN gene signature score to those with a positive QuantiFERON-TB Gold (QFT) test and unknown cause of uveitis. They concluded that a gene score of >5.61 showed high sensitivity (100%) and specificity (91%) for current TB infection and allowed to group patients into high or low risk for TB uveitis [51]. Such data show promising results for combining different strategies in our clinical practices, to reach a more reliable diagnosis.

To assess the effectiveness of chest X-rays (CXRs) in TB uveitis, Shaw et al. presented data from masked and independently reported CXRs by a pulmonologist and a radiologist. From a post hoc analysis on the results, it was calculated that CXR had a sensitivity, specificity, positive predictive value (PPV), and negative predictive value (NPV) of 14.7%, 94.3%, 55.6%, and 69.5%, respectively. They compared it with findings in those with intraocular sarcoidosis and reported a weak diagnostic accuracy of CXR in TB uveitis. However, CXRs are routinely done in the evaluation of those with presumed TB uveitis [52]. It can be suggested that local data should be utilized in deciding whether to perform CXR or not as validation of diagnostic tests varies with prevalence of systemic disease in local population (see **Figure 1**).

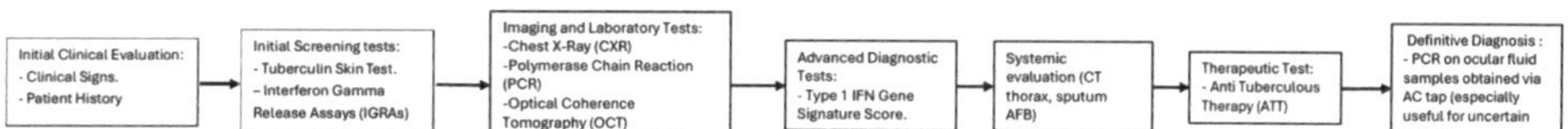

Figure 1.
Diagnostic algorithm summarizing approach to TB uveitis.

5. TB uveitis imaging

Various imaging modalities play a crucial role in TBU, given its diverse presentations. In classic cases, a fundoscopic exam alone can strongly suggest the diagnosis; however, newer and more advanced imaging techniques are increasingly being utilized to diagnose and document disease progression and treatment response. Digital imaging of the fundus allows documentation of clinical features of the disease and ultra-wide field (UWF) imaging permits imaging of the whole of the posterior segment [53]. UWF images record a 102–200 degrees view and are hence more useful in clinical decision-making for peripheral lesions [54]. Digital fundus imaging is often combined with fundus fluorescein angiography (FFA), which aids in the diagnosis of certain types of TB uveitis, differentiates active from inactive, and can also help in localizing complications, such as neovascularization, ischaemia, and macular oedema. FFA also plays a role in retinal vasculitis as it aids in visualization of phlebitis and other features of vasculitis.

Optical coherence tomography (OCT) is an important tool in the management of various retinal pathologies including TB uveitis and gives high-quality cross-sectional images of the retina and the retinal vasculature. Agarwal et al. discussed utilization of enhanced depth imaging (EDI) OCT, to evaluate structural changes that can be observed in cases with TB-SLC. They compared cases with controls and observed that the choroidal vascularity index (CVI) (calculated by dividing luminal area with total choroid area after processing image on the software: ImageJ (U.S. National Institutes of Health, Bethesda, MD, USA)) shows a significant decrease in those with tuberculous multifocal choroiditis (TB MFC), whereas choroidal thickness was greater [55].

OCT angiography (OCT-A) combines OCT with angiography and allows recording of retinal and choroidal vasculature. Areas or lesions with active disease show hypoperfusion on scans and complications, such as choroidal neovascularization (CNV), can be more easily detected [56]. OCT-A scans have shown to be sensitive in detecting blood flow impairment in choriocapillaris in TB-SLC. Serial OCT-A scans revealed atrophy of choriocapillaris in large TB SLC lesions as compared to healing after smaller lesions with restoration of perfusion in smaller lesions [57].

6. TB uveitis treatment

6.1 When to initiate ATT: Consensus guidelines

The Collaborative Ocular Tuberculosis Study (COTS) group identified clinical questions and asked 81 experts from all over the world to form agreement for initiating ATT in TB choroiditis using the Delphi process. Ten consensus statements out of 70 referring to the initiation of ATT in the three subtypes of TB choroiditis were established. It was decided that ATT could be started if positive results for any of the immunologic tests and radiologic findings suggestive of TB are present. For TB-SLC and tuberculoma, even a single positive immunologic test result, even in the absence of radiologic findings, was enough to start ATT [58]. A similar second guideline was published by the COTS group regarding ATT in TB anterior, intermediate, and panuveitis, and retinal vasculitis. Three hundred and twenty-four questions were initially included, which led to 44 consensus guidelines. It was agreed upon to start ATT in TB anterior uveitis (recurrent episodes) and other types of uveitis under study, if there is a positive result for any one of the immunologic tests and radiologic findings suggestive of TB. ATT was to be given only in cases where it is the first instance of TB anterior uveitis and if patients have inactive retinal vasculitis along with positive findings on radiological and immunological tests [59]. A Delphi survey similar to the COTS consensus guideline was performed by Basu et al. involving uveitis specialists from the Asia-Pacific region. The experts looked at various prognostic factors for the disease and concluded that time of disease, findings on imaging, prior steroid or immunosuppressant use, human immunodeficiency virus (HIV) infection, and multidrug-resistant tuberculosis (MDR-TB) are poor prognostic factors, whereas ATT for a period of more than 9 months was considered a positive prognostic feature [60]. Typically, treatment consists of a 4-drug anti-tubercular regimen (e.g., isoniazid, rifampicin, ethambutol, pyrazinamide) for 2 months, then extended treatment with isoniazid and rifampicin for another 6–12 months, in ocular TB due to its paucibacillary nature (see **Table 3**) [61]. Manousaridis et al. suggested at least 6 months of therapy and other experts favor longer courses [62].

The COTS group reported data of 945 patients from 25 international eye centers [63]. They looked at the regional variations in terms of disease management and outcomes, reporting poorer outcomes in those from Western countries. Ninety-two percent of the combined study population showed no symptoms and 76.7% had no history of pulmonary tuberculosis. Their data also showed that the biggest group of patients in all four regions under study received both anti-tuberculous treatment (ATT) and steroids. However, high treatment failure rates in this group of patients could suggest that both ATT and steroids were prescribed to patients with refractory or difficult-to-manage disease. This indicates that those given dual treatment with ATT and steroids had severe disease to begin with, which resulted in higher treatment failure rates. One hundred and eighty-nine patients out of the total 702 (26.9%) with chest X-rays (CXRs) available showed a pulmonary lesion; on the other hand, 109 patients out of the total 159 (68.6%) of those with computed tomography (CT) of thorax were positive for a pulmonary finding. This shows a higher sensitivity of CT thorax for picking up pulmonary disease, but higher costs and radiation compared to CXR discourage its use for screening purposes.

Therapy modality	Role in TBU management
Anti-tubercular therapy (ATT)	Mainstay treatment for TBU, targeting the underlying *Mycobacterium tuberculosis* infection. Indicated for all presumed or confirmed TB uveitis cases.
Systemic corticosteroids	Indicated in all cases to control inflammation especially if vision-threatening, often in conjunction with ATT.
Systemic immunosuppressants	Employed in cases with severe inflammation or when corticosteroids are insufficient. For steroid-sparing in chronic cases or if paradoxical inflammation occurs. Examples include: azathioprine, methotrexate, and mycophenolate. Caution: To be used only after excluding active TB and in consultation with infectious disease specialists.
Intravitreal therapy	Include intravitreal dexamethasone and methotrexate for local control of inflammation and anti-VEGF injections for neovascular complications.
Laser/vitrectomy	Utilized for managing complications, such as retinal detachment (laser for rhegmatogenous retinal detachment (RRD) and vitrectomy for tractional retinal detachment (TRD)), non-resolving vitreous haze or persistent vitreous hemorrhage. Laser to be used for ischaemic vasculitis/proliferative retinopathy.

Table 3.
Treatment modalities for TB uveitis.

In practice, if clinical suspicion remains exceedingly high (e.g., progressive serpiginous-like choroiditis) despite negative laboratory tests, many experts advocate a trial of ATT after other diagnoses (like sarcoidosis) are reasonably excluded. This approach is controversial but can be considered in sight-threatening scenarios, as delaying treatment may lead to irreversible damage.

6.2 Outcomes of treatment: Evidence from endemic vs. non-endemic regions

A prospective study was conducted at a large tertiary care center in Karachi, Pakistan, which has one of the highest TB incidences in the world [64]. Ghauri et al. reviewed 40 patients for TB uveitis, with 90% of the cases diagnosed with posterior uveitis. They reported resolution of disease in 80% of the patients after 12 months of ATT and steroids were given to three patients who developed acute vitritis. Their experience in a high-burden setting underscores that TB should be considered in any uveitis case in endemic areas, and prompt work-up (and treatment) should be undertaken to confirm and address TB as the cause. Hong Kong is another TB-endemic region and in a case series from year 2000 to 2015 Chung et al. used positive T-SPOT.TB as a confirmation for TB uveitis [65]. Twenty-five of the 75 patients tested came out positive and 14 were started on ATT. Seven patients were later started on systemic steroids and one patient underwent vitrectomy for vitritis. At the end of 1 year, 92.9% of the cases achieved remission and only three were given steroids beyond this period. Tsui et al. reported outcomes of patients with TB uveitis in their hospital in Hong Kong over a period of 2014–2019. As many as 94.7% of their study participants were given ATT and 94.4% were given a combination of ATT and steroids [66]. Moreover, 31.6% of the 19 participants were started on immunosuppressants before ATT was started. They reported an overall improvement in patients treated with this approach, except for those with intermediate uveitis as all of them showed worsened signs of inflammation. TB retinal vasculitis was the most common presentation in their setting (42.1%) and required treatment with a combination of ATT and steroids. Good clinical results from ATT in patients from endemic regions as seen in these studies provide evidence for its utility in populations with extensive BCG vaccination coverage.

Tomkins-Netzer et al. present data from two non-endemic regions of patients with uveitis and latent TB infection. They had a sample of 129 patients and concluded that those treated with ATT (29.5%) had a lower recurrence rate as compared to those who were not (48.2%). ATT also showed benefit, in the sense that it delayed recurrence in those who did develop it [67]. In another non-endemic TB area, Manousaridis et al. concluded that at least 6 months of ATT in either confirmed or presumed cases of TB as a cause of uveitis provides good clinical results [62]. Ninety percent of their 24 patients received ATT, whereas 20% received systemic steroids. Pars plana vitrectomy was done in two patients for diagnostic purpose and for clearing a vitreous hemorrhage, respectively.

In TB-endemic regions, clinicians may encounter patients with uveitis who have undergone positive TB tests by virtue of latent infection rather than actual ocular TB. In such cases, a careful work-up to exclude other causes (e.g., sarcoidosis, viral uveitis) is crucial. If no alternative cause is found, many experts would still initiate ATT given the high prevalence of TB and potential benefits as shown by studies, but this must be an individualized decision [67].

6.3 Complications and their management

Common complications associated with TB uveitis include cataract formation, glaucoma, cystoid macular oedema (CME), vitreous hemorrhage, tractional retinal detachment from vasculitis, and choroidal neovascularization (CNV). Cataract may result from chronic uveitis or prolonged corticosteroid use and is typically managed with cataract surgery, once the inflammation is well controlled. Glaucoma frequently arises secondary to uveitis or steroid therapy; intraocular pressure (IOP) should be regularly monitored, with elevated IOP managed using IOP-lowering therapy or surgical intervention, as needed. CNV is typically addressed with intravitreal anti-VEGF injections. In cases of non-clearing vitreous hemorrhage or for diagnostic biopsy, pars plana vitrectomy may be indicated. Effective identification and timely management of these complications are essential for preserving vision in patients with uveitis.

6.4 Intravitreal dexamethasone

ATT is considered the mainstay of treatment in TB uveitis with concurrent steroid and immunosuppressants often needed to control paradoxical worsening of inflammation seen with onset of ATT regimen. High-dose systemic steroids are sometimes needed to achieve high enough dose in the posterior segment, which cannot be continued for longer periods of time due to the concern of developing various side effects. In such cases, intravitreal dexamethasone implants can be used. Jain et al. reviewed the efficacy of using such implants (Ozurdex) in six patients with multifocal serpiginoid choroiditis [29]. Half of these patients received Ozurdex for worsening intraocular inflammation and the other half due to contraindications to systemic therapy. Six of the six patients had complete recovery within approximately 9 weeks on average, which shows good supporting evidence of its use. Agarwal et al. report their patient's response to intravitreal dexamethasone implants with concomitant ATT. In a retrospective series of 17 TB uveitis patients treated with Ozurdex implants alongside ATT, all showed improved inflammation and vision (see **Table 4**) [68].

6.5 Intravitreal methotrexate

Intravitreal methotrexate (IVT MTX) is a form of local immunosuppression, which is sometimes considered in cases with poor response to treatments already discussed above. Three eyes in two patients in a study by Julain et al. were given IVT MTX and showed healing of lesions within a month and helped in controlling local inflammation where systemic ATT had not succeeded [69]. Another case is reported by Tsui et al., in which the patient had previously been treated with ATT for serpiginous-like choroiditis 2 years before developing a new lesion [70]. She was started on

Therapy	Use in TBU	Evidence	Remarks
Ozurdex	Severe posterior uveitis	Jain et al. and Agarwal et al. reported improvement in all 6 and 17 of their patients, respectively.	Avoids systemic side effects; monitor for intraocular pressure rise
IVT methotrexate	Refractory serpiginous-like choroiditis	Case reports with lesion healing. Off-label use of intravitreal methotrexate for refractory cases.	Last-resort, experimental option
Anti-VEGF	Retinal/choroidal neovascular complications	Case reports including one successful monotherapy.	Adjunct therapy to reduce tuberculous lesions with high vascularity.

Table 4.
Intravitreal treatment modalities.

ATT, steroids, and immunosuppressant drugs simultaneously but still showed worsening of disease. IVT MTX was then given in two divided doses 1 month apart and the lesions regressed, and inflammation subsided. The use of IVT MTX is still novel and unconventional but shows potential as a last resort in the difficult-to-treat cases.

6.6 Intravitreal anti-VEGF

A few cases in the literature have been described where intravitreal anti-VEGF injections helped in the treatment of vascular TB choroidal granulomas, often alongside systemic ATT, and steroids. However, Jain et al. managed to treat a case of choroidal tuberculoma with just intravitreal ranibizumab with regression of the disease within 6 weeks without recurrence and significant visual recovery [71]. Hence, it shows the utility of intravitreal anti-VEGF injections in tuberculous lesions with high vascularity.

If intraocular inflammation remains severe, despite systemic ATT and steroid therapy (or if systemic therapy is contraindicated), an intravitreal dexamethasone implant can be considered to achieve local disease control. Intravitreal methotrexate may be reserved for refractory cases that fail both ATT and conventional immunosuppression. Anti-VEGF is primarily used for complications like choroidal neovascular membranes or persistent vascular leakage but may also have a role in treating choroidal lesions with high angiogenic activity.

7. Limitations and real-world obstacles

Several clinically challenging scenarios have been addressed in this chapter, including diagnostic ambiguity while dealing with TB uveitis cases, especially in TB-endemic regions with high latent TB prevalence. This challenge is further exacerbated by lack of a single gold standard test for TB uveitis. However, a systematic diagnostic and treatment approach as outlined above helps in managing majority of the cases. Furthermore, IGRA remains positive even after treatment, so in endemic areas or treated cases, results need clinical and radiologic context.

TB is highly prevalent in developing parts of the world with a high burden of disease in areas like South Asia. In these resource-limited settings, delays in diagnosis are often faced due to lack of access to advanced diagnostic tests. Another challenge faced in these settings is unavailability of newer, promising therapies. Lastly, management challenges include deciding the optimal duration of anti-tubercular therapy (ATT), steroid use, and addressing paradoxical reactions—each requiring careful clinical judgment on a case-by-case basis.

8. Conclusion

Tuberculosis (TB) has a high global burden of disease, making TB uveitis a crucial yet frequently under-recognized cause of uveitis. TBU presents with diverse phenotypes, lacks a definitive diagnostic test, and requires a high index of suspicion. Diagnostic strategies should be individualized based on regional TB prevalence and clinical presentation, integrating IGRA, imaging, and therapeutic response. Emerging diagnostics, including gene expression profiling and OCT angiography, alongside new therapeutic modalities such as intravitreal methotrexate and anti-VEGF, offer hope for better individualized care. Incorporating guideline-based, context-sensitive management approaches into clinical practice can improve visual outcomes and reduce diagnostic delay in this under-recognized cause of uveitis. Ongoing research into more accurate diagnostics and targeted therapies holds promise to further improve the care of TBU patients.

Author details

Roha Ahmad Choudhary
The Aga Khan University, Karachi, Pakistan

*Address all correspondence to: rohaahmedchoudhary@yahoo.com

References

[1] World Health Organization. Global tuberculosis control: Key findings from the December 2009 WHO report. Weekly Epidemiological Record= Relevé épidémiologique hebdomadaire. 2010;**85**(09):69-79

[2] Varma D, Anand S, Reddy AR, Das A, Watson JP, Currie DC, et al. Tuberculosis: An under-diagnosed aetiological agent in uveitis with an effective treatment. Eye. 2006;**20**(9):1068-1073

[3] Helm CJ, Holland GN. Ocular tuberculosis. Survey of Ophthalmology. 1993;**38**:229-256

[4] Houben RM, Dodd PJ. The global burden of latent tuberculosis infection: A re-estimation using mathematical modelling. PLoS Medicine. 2016;**13**(10):e1002152

[5] World Health Organization. Global Tuberculosis Report 2020. Geneva: World Health Organization; 2020

[6] Shakarchi FI. Ocular tuberculosis: Current perspectives. Clinical Ophthalmology (Auckland, NZ). 2015;**9**:2223

[7] Cunningham ET, Rathinam SR, Albini TA, Chee SP, Zierhut M. Tuberculous uveitis. Ocular Immunology and Inflammation. 2015;**23**(1):2-6

[8] Tagirasa R, Parmar S, Barik MR, Devadas S, Basu S. Autoreactive T cells in immunopathogenesis of TB-associated uveitis. Investigative Ophthalmology and Visual Science. 2017;**58**(13):5682-5691

[9] Ishaq M, Muhammad JS, Mahmood K. Uveitis is not just an ophthalmologists' concern. JPMA. Journal of the Pakistan Medical Association. 2012;**62**(2):92

[10] Rosenbaum JT. To be or not TB? British Journal of Ophthalmology. 2014;**98**:999-1000

[11] Hong BK, Khanamiri HN, Bababeygy SR, Rao NA. The utility of routine tuberculosis screening in county hospital patients with uveitis. British Journal of Ophthalmology. 2014;**98**(8):1091-1095

[12] Patel SS, Saraiya NV, Tessler HH, Goldstein DA. Mycobacterial ocular inflammation: Delay in diagnosis and other factors impacting morbidity. JAMA Ophthalmology. 2013;**131**(6):752-758

[13] Al-Qarni A, Abouammoh MA, Almousa AN, Mousa A, Abu El-Asrar AM. Presumed tuberculous uveitis in a university-based tertiary referral center in Saudi Arabia. International Ophthalmology. 2019;**39**(2):317-333

[14] Mao Y, Peng XY, You QS, Wang H, Zhao M, Jonas JB. Tuberculous uveitis in China. Acta Ophthalmologica. 2014;**92**(5):e393-e397

[15] Krassas N, Wells J, Bell C, Woodhead M, Jones N. Presumed tuberculosis-associated uveitis: Rising incidence and widening criteria for diagnosis in a non-endemic area. Eye. 2018;**32**(1):87-92

[16] Shirley K, Dowlut S, Silvestri J, Pavesio C, Foot B. Presumed ocular tuberculosis in the United Kingdom: A British ophthalmological surveillance unit (BOSU) study. Eye. 2020;**34**(10):1835-1841

[17] Ng KK, Nisbet M, Damato EM, Sims JL. Presumed tuberculous uveitis in non-endemic country for tuberculosis:

Case series from a New Zealand tertiary uveitis clinic. Clinical and Experimental Ophthalmology. 2017;**45**(4):357-365

[18] Institute of Environmental Science and Research Ltd. Tuberculosis in New Zealand: Annual Report 2014. Porirua, New Zealand: Institute of Environmental Science and Research Ltd; 2015

[19] Darian-Smith E, Lin ML, Lim LL, McCluskey P, Hall AJ. The incidence of ocular tuberculosis in Australia over the past 10 years (2006-2015). Ophthalmic Epidemiology. 2017;**24**(6):406-412

[20] Figueira L, Fonseca S, Ladeira I, Duarte R. Ocular tuberculosis: Position paper on diagnosis and treatment management. Revista Portuguesa de Pneumologia (English Edition). 2017;**23**(1):31-38

[21] Ang M, Wong WL, Kiew SY, Li X, Chee SP. Prospective head-to-head study comparing 2 commercial interferon gamma release assays for the diagnosis of tuberculous uveitis. American Journal of Ophthalmology. 2014;**157**(6):1306-1314.e4

[22] Gupta A, Sharma A, Bansal R, Sharma K. Classification of intraocular tuberculosis. Ocular Immunology and Inflammation. 2015;**23**(1):7-13

[23] Gupta V, Gupta A, Rao NA. Intraocular tuberculosis—An update. Survey of Ophthalmology. 2007;**52**(6):561-587

[24] Gupta V, Shoughy SS, Mahajan S, Khairallah M, Rosenbaum JT, Curi A, et al. Clinics of ocular tuberculosis. Ocular Immunology and Inflammation. 2015;**23**(1):14-24

[25] Mehta S, Banker AS, Chauhan R. Retinal and choroidal manifestations of tuberculosis. In: Retinal and Choroidal Manifestations of Selected Systemic Diseases. New York, NY: Springer New York; 15 Jun 2012. pp. 63-78

[26] Ness T, Boehringer D, Heinzelmann S. Intermediate uveitis: Pattern of etiology, complications, treatment and outcome in a tertiary academic center. Orphanet Journal of Rare Diseases. 2017;**12**:81

[27] Babu K, Bhat SS. Unilateral snow banking in tuberculosis-related intermediate uveitis. Journal of Ophthalmic Inflammation and Infection. 2014;**4**(1):4

[28] Gan WL, Jones NP. Serpiginous-like choroiditis as a marker for tuberculosis in a non-endemic area. British Journal of Ophthalmology. 2013;**97**(5):644-647

[29] Jain L, Panda KG, Basu S. Clinical outcomes of adjunctive sustained-release intravitreal dexamethasone implants in tuberculosis-associated multifocal serpigenoid choroiditis. Ocular Immunology and Inflammation. 2018;**26**(6):877-883

[30] Bansal R, Gupta A, Gupta V, Dogra MR, Sharma A, Bambery P. Tubercular serpiginous-like choroiditis presenting as multifocal serpiginoid choroiditis. Ophthalmology. 2012;**119**(11):2334-2342

[31] Agarwal A, Marchese A, Rabiolo A, Agrawal R, Bansal R, Gupta V. Clinical and imaging factors associated with the outcomes of tubercular serpiginous-like choroiditis. American Journal of Ophthalmology. 2020;**220**:160-169

[32] Zhang M, Zhang J, Liu Y. Clinical presentations and therapeutic effect of presumed choroidal tuberculosis. Retina. 2012;**32**(4):805-813

[33] Pathanapitoon K, Rothova A, Apinyawasisuk S, Kunavisarut P. Clinical

features and etiology of retinal vasculitis in Northern Thailand. Indian Journal of Ophthalmology. 2013;**61**(12):739

[34] Das T, Pathengay A, Hussain N, Biswas J. Eales' disease: Diagnosis and management. Eye. 2010;**24**(3):472-482

[35] Patricio MS, Portelinha J, Passarinho MP, Guedes ME. Tubercular retinal vasculitis. Case Reports. 2013;**2013**:bcr2013008924

[36] Khan MN, Raza SS, Qadir S, Rehman H, Hussain AK, Nadeem MD, et al. Eales disease. Journal of Ayub Medical College, Abbottabad. 2016;**28**(4):816-817

[37] Madhavan HN, Therese KL, Doraiswamy K. Further investigations on the association of *Mycobacterium tuberculosis* with Eales' disease. Indian Journal of Ophthalmology. 2002;**50**(1):35-39

[38] Therese KL, Deepa P, Therese J, Bagyalakshmi R, Biswas J, Madhavan HN. Association of mycobacteria with Eales' disease. The Indian Journal of Medical Research. 2007;**126**(1):56-62

[39] Singh R, Toor P, Parchand S, Sharma K, Gupta V, Gupta A. Quantitative polymerase chain reaction for *Mycobacterium tuberculosis* in so-called Eales' disease. Ocular Immunology and Inflammation. 2012;**20**(3):153-157

[40] Pai M, Denkinger CM, Kik SV, Rangaka MX, Zwerling A, Oxlade O, et al. Gamma interferon release assays for detection of *Mycobacterium tuberculosis* infection. Clinical Microbiology Reviews. 2014;**27**(1):3-20

[41] Ang M, Vasconcelos-Santos DV, Sharma K, Accorinti M, Sharma A, Gupta A, et al. Diagnosis of ocular tuberculosis. Ocular Immunology and Inflammation. 2018;**26**(2):208-216

[42] Lou SM, Montgomery PA, Larkin KL, Winthrop K, Zierhut M, Rosenbaum JT, et al. Diagnosis and treatment for ocular tuberculosis among uveitis specialists: The international perspective. Ocular Immunology and Inflammation. 2015;**23**(1):32-39

[43] Rahman S, Irfan M, Siddiqui MR. Role of interferon gamma release assay in the diagnosis and management of Mycobacterium tuberculosis-associated uveitis: A review. BMJ Open Ophthalmology. 2021;**6**(1):e000663

[44] Masae Kawamura L. QuantiFERON-TB Gold Plus the 4th Generation IGRA [Internet]. 2017. Available from: https://www.who.int/tb/areas-of-work/preventive-care/ltbi/mk.pdf?ua=1

[45] Barcellini L, Borroni E, Brown J, Brunetti E, Codecasa L, Cugnata F, et al. First independent evaluation of QuantiFERON-TB plus performance. European Respiratory Journal. 2016;**47**(5):1587-1590

[46] Takeda K, Nagai H, Suzukawa M, Sekiguchi R, Akashi S, Sato R, et al. Comparison of QuantiFERON-TB gold plus, QuantiFERON-TB gold in-tube, and T-SPOT. TB among patients with tuberculosis. Journal of Infection and Chemotherapy. 2020;**26**(11):1205-1212

[47] Nora RLD, Putera I, Khalisha DF, Septiana I, Sitompul R. The diagnostic value of polymerase chain reaction for ocular tuberculosis diagnosis in relation to antitubercular therapy response: A meta-analysis. International Journal of Infectious Diseases. 2021;**110**:394-402

[48] Agarwal A, Agrawal R, Gunasekaran DV, Raje D, Gupta B,

Aggarwal K, et al. The collaborative ocular tuberculosis study (COTS)-1 report 3: Polymerase chain reaction in the diagnosis and management of tubercular uveitis: Global trends. Ocular Immunology and Inflammation. 2019;**27**(3):465-473

[49] Ludi Z, Sule AA, Samy RP, Putera I, Schrijver B, Hutchinson PE, et al. Diagnosis and biomarkers for ocular tuberculosis: From the present into the future. Theranostics. 2023;**13**(7):2088-2113

[50] Sharma K, Sharma M, Ayyadurai N, Dogra M, Sharma A, Gupta V, et al. Comparative evaluation of GeneXpert MTB/RIF ultra and GeneXpert MTB/RIF for detecting tuberculosis and identifying rifampicin resistance in pars Plana vitrectomy samples of patients with ocular tuberculosis. Ocular Immunology and Inflammation. 2023;**31**(5):914-920

[51] La Distia NR, Sitompul R, Bakker M, Versnel MA, Swagemakers SM, van der Spek PJ, et al. Type 1 interferon-inducible gene expression in QuantiFERON Gold TB-positive uveitis: A tool to stratify a high versus low risk of active tuberculosis? PLoS ONE. 2018;**13**(10):e0206073

[52] Shaw JA, Smit DP, Griffith-Richards S, Koegelenberg CFN. Utility of routine chest radiography in ocular tuberculosis and sarcoidosis. The International Journal of Tuberculosis and Lung Disease. 2018;**22**(11):1374-1377

[53] Bansal R, Basu S, Gupta A, Rao N, Invernizzi A, Kramer M. Imaging in tuberculosis-associated uveitis. Indian Journal of Ophthalmology. 2017;**65**(4):264

[54] Aggarwal K, Mulkutkar S, Mahajan S, Singh R, Sharma A, Bansal R, et al. Role of ultra-wide field imaging in the management of tubercular posterior uveitis. Ocular Immunology and Inflammation. 2016;**24**(6):631-636

[55] Agarwal A, Agrawal R, Khandelwal N, Invernizzi A, Aggarwal K, Sharma A, et al. Choroidal structural changes in tubercular multifocal serpiginoid choroiditis. Ocular Immunology and Inflammation. 2018;**26**(6):838-844

[56] Aggarwal K, Agarwal A, Sharma A, Sharma K, Gupta V, OCTA Study Group. Detection of type 1 choroidal neovascular membranes using optical coherence tomography angiography in tubercular posterior uveitis. Retina. 2019;**39**(8):1595-1606

[57] Agarwal A, Aggarwal K, Mandadi SKR, Kumar A, Grewal D, Invernizzi A, et al. Longitudinal follow-up of tubercular serpiginous-like choroiditis using optical coherence tomography angiography. Retina. 2021;**41**(4):793-803

[58] Agrawal R, Testi I, Mahajan S, Yuen YS, Agarwal A, Kon OM, et al. Collaborative Ocular Tuberculosis Study consensus guidelines on the management of tubercular uveitis—Report 1: Guidelines for initiating antitubercular therapy in tubercular choroiditis. Ophthalmology. 2021;**128**(2):266-276

[59] Agrawal R, Testi I, Bodaghi B, Barisani-Asenbauer T, McCluskey P, Agarwal A, et al. Collaborative Ocular Tuberculosis Study consensus guidelines on the management of tubercular uveitis—Report 2: Guidelines for initiating antitubercular therapy in anterior uveitis, intermediate uveitis, panuveitis, and retinal vasculitis. Ophthalmology. 2021;**128**(2):277-287

[60] Basu S, Nora RLD, Rao NA, Jiang X, Fuady A. Prognostic factors for

TB-associated uveitis in the Asia-Pacific Region: Results of a modified Delphi survey. Eye. 2020;**34**(9):1693-1701

[61] Akhavanrezayat A, Uludag Kirimli G, Matsumiya W, Khojasteh H, Or C, Karaca I, et al. The role of corticosteroids and immunomodulatory therapy in the management of infectious uveitis. Ocular Immunology and Inflammation. 2024;**32**(8):1832-1843

[62] Manousaridis K, Ong E, Stenton C, Gupta R, Browning AC, Pandit R. Clinical presentation, treatment, and outcomes in presumed intraocular tuberculosis: Experience from Newcastle upon Tyne, UK. Eye. 2013;**27**(4):480-486

[63] Agrawal R, Gunasekeran DV, Raje D, Agarwal A, Nguyen QD, Kon OM, et al. Global variations and challenges with tubercular uveitis in the collaborative ocular tuberculosis study. Investigative Ophthalmology and Visual Science. 2018;**59**(10):4162-4171

[64] Ghauri MI, Iqbal N, Riaz SU, Irfan M, Kumar A, Mukarram MS. Visual and treatment outcomes of tubercular uveitis: A prospective case series from a referral hospital in Pakistan. BMC Research Notes. 2019;**12**(1):1-4

[65] Chung CY, Li KK. The efficacy of latent tuberculosis treatment for immunocompetent uveitis patients with a positive T-SPOT. TB test: 6-year experience in a tuberculosis endemic region. International Ophthalmology. 2018;**38**(6):2273-2282

[66] Tsui J, Ho M, Lui G, Li T, Chen L, Iu L, et al. The clinical presentation and treatment outcomes of ocular tuberculosis: A 5-year experience in an endemic area. International Ophthalmology. Sep 2021;**41**(9):3199-3209

[67] Tomkins-Netzer O, Leong BC, Zhang X, Lightman S, McCluskey PJ, Lee AJ, et al. Effect of antituberculous therapy on uveitis associated with latent tuberculosis. American Journal of Ophthalmology. 2018;**190**:164-170

[68] Agarwal A, Handa S, Aggarwal K, Sharma M, Singh R, Sharma A, et al. The role of dexamethasone implant in the management of tubercular uveitis. Ocular Immunology and Inflammation. 2018;**26**(6):884-892

[69] Julian K, Langner-Wegscheider BJ, Haas A, De Smet MD. Intravitreal methotrexate in the management of presumed tuberculous serpiginous-like choroiditis. Retina. 2013;**33**(9):1943-1948

[70] Tsui E, Fern CM, Goldberg NR. Treatment of refractory tubercular serpiginous–like choroiditis with intravitreal methotrexate. Retinal Cases and Brief Reports. 2021;**15**(2):169-173

[71] Jain S, Agarwal A, Gupta V. Resolution of large choroidal tuberculoma following monotherapy with intravitreal ranibizumab. Ocular Immunology and Inflammation. 2 Apr 2020

Chapter 4

Clinical Features and Treatment Options of Vogt-Koyanagi-Harada Disease

Mustafa Kayabaşı

Abstract

Vogt-Koyanagi-Harada (VKH) disease is a rare, multisystem autoimmune disorder targeting melanocyte-rich tissues, such as the uveal tract, meninges, inner ear, skin, and hair. Ocular involvement, typically presenting as bilateral granulomatous panuveitis with exudative retinal detachment, represents the hallmark manifestation and often precedes systemic features, such as meningismus, tinnitus, alopecia, poliosis, and vitiligo. Diagnosis is based on clinical criteria, supported by advanced imaging modalities, including optical coherence tomography, indocyanine green angiography, and fundus autofluorescence, which enable precise evaluation of choroidal inflammation and treatment response. Early, high-dose corticosteroid therapy remains the cornerstone of treatment, often combined with immunosuppressive agents to prevent chronic complications, such as sunset glow fundus, cataract, and subretinal fibrosis. Biological therapies have emerged as effective options for refractory or chronic cases. Advances in imaging and immunopathogenic understanding have significantly enhanced the diagnostic and therapeutic approach to VKH disease. Future advancements in the management of VKH disease may include the development of novel targeted therapies and the integration of advanced imaging techniques. Additionally, artificial intelligence may also play a role in enhancing early detection of the disease, personalizing treatment approaches, and improving the prognosis.

Keywords: corticosteroids, granulomatous panuveitis, ocular inflammation, optical coherence tomography, uveo-meningeal syndrome, Vogt-Koyanagi-Harada disease

1. Introduction

Vogt-Koyanagi-Harada (VKH) disease is a multisystem autoimmune disorder that primarily targets melanocyte-containing tissues. It is most notably characterized by bilateral granulomatous posterior uveitis, which may progress to involve the entire uveal tract. In addition to ocular findings, the syndrome frequently presents with neurologic symptoms, such as tinnitus, vertigo, or sensorineural hearing loss, due to involvement of the eighth cranial nerve. Dermatologic manifestations, including vitiligo, alopecia, and poliosis, often appear in later stages of the disease and reflect the systemic nature of the autoimmune response. The clinical spectrum and disease course may vary, but prompt diagnosis and immunosuppressive therapy are essential to prevent irreversible visual and systemic complications [1, 2].

The initial description of VKH disease dates back to 1906, when Vogt [3] reported a case of nontraumatic uveitis accompanied by poliosis. In 1929, Koyanagi [4] documented patients with bilateral idiopathic uveitis associated with systemic manifestations, such as poliosis, vitiligo, dysacousia, and alopecia. Due to the consistent clinical presentation among these cases, the condition was subsequently recognized as a distinct uveitic entity and referred to as Vogt–Koyanagi syndrome [5]. Separately, in 1926, Harada [6] described a form of uveitis characterized by cerebrospinal fluid (CSF) pleocytosis and serous retinal detachment, which was initially considered a different disease entity. However, accumulating evidence over the years has indicated that Vogt–Koyanagi syndrome and Harada disease represent different clinical phases of the same underlying disorder [7].

The estimated incidence rate stands at about 15 per million people [8]. The prevalence of VKH disease varies by region, with a higher frequency among women in North America. In contrast, men are more commonly affected in Japan. Additionally, VKH is more prevalent in Japan, where it represents 10.1% of all uveitis cases, compared to just 7% of uveitis referrals in the United States [9]. In contrast, countries like Brazil and Colombia report a lower prevalence of VKH, with the disease accounting for 6 and 1.2%, respectively, of all uveitis cases [10]. Although VKH primarily affects individuals between the ages of 20 and 50, it has also been reported in children [11]. The occurrence of VKH disease also shows notable variation across different ethnic groups. It is more commonly observed among individuals with darker pigmentation, such as Asians, Hispanics, Native Americans, and people of South Asian descent. In contrast, the condition appears to be relatively rare among Caucasians and individuals of sub-Saharan African origin [1].

The exact pathogenesis of VKH disease remains incompletely understood. However, it is widely believed that microbial infections may serve as environmental triggers, initiating an autoimmune response in genetically susceptible individuals. This immune response appears to target several ocular antigens, including melanin-associated antigens, interphotoreceptor retinoid-binding protein, and retinal S-antigen, ultimately contributing to the development and progression of the disease [12]. Historically, VKH disease has been primarily characterized as a non-necrotizing, diffuse granulomatous inflammation of the uveal tract, bearing histopathological similarities to sympathetic ophthalmia [13]. Histopathological studies have shown that in VKH disease, inflammation primarily targets the choroid—autoimmune reaction against tyrosinase-like proteins in melanocytes in the uvea —while retinal involvement tends to occur later, likely as a secondary effect. In the early stage of VKH disease, the choriocapillaris, the retinal pigment epithelium (RPE), and the neurosensory retina are typically spared, possibly due in part to the immunomodulatory role of RPE cells in suppressing intraocular inflammation [14]. As the initial site of inflammation is the choroidal stroma within the uvea in VKH disease, it is referred to as primary stromal choroiditis [15].

Genetic associations, particularly with human leukocyte antigens DR4 (HLA-DR4) and DRw53 (HLA-DRw53), have been recognized in VKH disease [7]. There is growing evidence that various T-cell subsets, including Th17, Th1, and regulatory T (Treg) cells, along with their associated cytokines, such as interleukin-17 (IL-17), interferon-gamma (IFN-γ), tumor necrosis factor-alpha (TNF-α), IL-10, and transforming growth factor-beta (TGF-β), play a critical role in both the initiation and maintenance of the autoimmune response in VKH disease [13]. Recent studies also highlighted the involvement of IL-23 in the inflammatory cascade. This pathway contributes to the differentiation of Th17 cells and the subsequent production of IL-17, which plays a critical role in the disease's pathogenesis [2].

2. Clinical features

Vogt-Koyanagi-Harada disease is characterized by a spectrum of clinical manifestations that evolve throughout its course. Traditionally, the disease has been classified into four distinct stages: the prodromal stage, the acute uveitic stage, the chronic convalescent stage, and the chronic recurrent stage [16, 17]. However, more recently, VKH disease has been broadly categorized into two main stages: the early stage, encompassing the prodromal and acute uveitic phases, and the late stage, which includes the convalescent and chronic recurrent phases [15]. Each phase exhibits specific clinical features, underscoring the dynamic and progressive nature of the disease.

2.1 Early stage (prodromal, acute uveitic)

Patients with VKH disease often present with prodromal symptoms prior to the onset of overt ocular manifestations, including headache, nausea, low-grade fever, vertigo, tinnitus, signs of meningeal irritation, scalp tenderness, and periorbital pain [18]. Headache is the most frequently reported neurological symptom during the prodromal phase of Vogt-Koyanagi-Harada disease [19]. The prodromal phase of VKH disease generally lasts from several hours to a few days, though it can occasionally persist for weeks. During this period, subclinical choroiditis or meningeal inflammation may be present and can be detected by CSF analysis [15, 20]. Pleocytosis detected in CSF analysis is regarded as a characteristic finding in the early stages of VKH disease [17]. Although it is generally accepted that ocular involvement is absent during the prodromal phase of VKH disease, there have been reports documenting subclinical choroiditis and optic nerve involvement during this early stage [15, 21].

The disease becomes clinically manifest after the initial prodromal period. Sudden bilateral visual blurring and decreased visual acuity are the most common presenting symptoms in this phase. The majority of patients experience simultaneous vision loss in both eyes. Although one eye may be affected initially, 94% of cases will involve the second eye within 2 weeks [19].

Diffuse choroiditis followed by bilateral, granulomatous posterior uveitis represents the hallmark clinical presentation of VKH disease during this stage. Primary choroidal inflammation can secondarily affect adjacent ocular structures, including the optic disc, retina, ciliary body, and, in some cases, the anterior chamber [15]. In the acute phase of VKH disease, the formation of full-thickness granulomas can obstruct normal choroidal circulation. This leads to delayed filling of the choroidal arteries, followed by impaired perfusion of the choriocapillaris. The resulting reduction in blood supply is thought to cause acute ischemic injury, which may, in turn, contribute to the development of exudative retinal detachment [22]. Key features of posterior segment involvement in the acute stage include thickening of the posterior choroid, elevation of the peripapillary retinochoroidal layer, multiple exudative retinal detachments, and optic nerve head involvement, commonly manifesting as hyperemia and edema [7]. Optic nerve involvement is frequently observed during the acute stage of VKH disease, with optic nerve head swelling occurring in approximately 87% of patients [23]. Fluorescein angiography (FA) typically demonstrates optic disc leakage, or "hot disc," in around 94% of cases [24]. Retinal edema, another early sign of the disease, may be observed in the posterior pole. As the disease progresses, exudative retinal detachment, a key diagnostic feature, may develop, with the inferior portion of the retina being most frequently involved. In the retinal periphery, yellow-white, well-circumscribed lesions may appear, resembling those seen in sympathetic ophthalmia. These lesions were previously believed to represent the clinical equivalent of Dalen-Fuchs nodules (**Figure 1**) [25].

In the absence of appropriate treatment at this stage, the inflammation often progresses anteriorly. Over time, it becomes more diffuse, eventually involving the anterior chamber and manifesting as panuveitis [26, 27]. Anterior segment manifestations of VKH disease are characterized by a granulomatous inflammatory response, with the presence of mutton-fat keratic precipitates on the corneal endothelium. Perilimbal vitiligo, also known as Sugiura sign, is a notable feature, occurring in approximately 85% of the patients [23]. Inflammatory activity can be severe, often involving both the anterior chamber and the anterior vitreous in around 56% of cases. Nodules may also be observed on the pupillary margin and within the iris stroma [19]. An early manifestation of the disease may include shallowing of the anterior chamber and a moderate increase in intraocular pressure. In cases of severe inflammation, the ciliary body may become involved, leading to the production of supraciliary fluid. This change is typically detected only through careful gonioscopic examination. The fluid accumulates at the site of ciliary detachment, resulting in myopic shift and, in some cases, angle-closure glaucoma [28, 29]. In contrast, some patients may present with hypotony, likely due to edema of the ciliary body [30, 31].

Tinnitus and hearing loss are the most common extraocular manifestations during the anterior uveal involvement stage. Although uncommon, integumentary changes, such as poliosis, alopecia, and vitiligo, may also be observed in some patients [7].

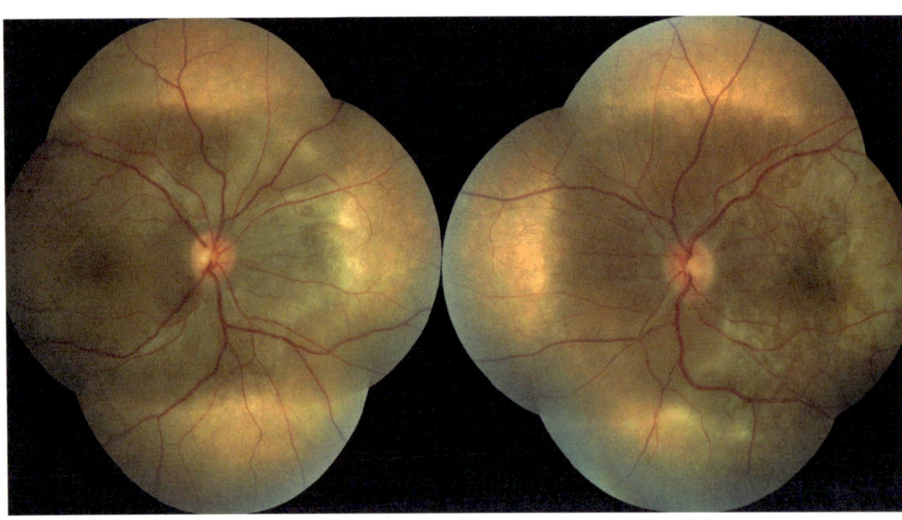

Figure 1.
Color fundus images of a patient with early-stage Vogt-Koyanagi-Harada disease showing bilateral extensive exudative retinal detachments accompanied by optic disc hyperemia at the posterior pole (Courtesy of Ali Osman Saatci, MD).

2.2 Late stage (convalescent, chronic recurrent)

Delaying or inadequately initiating appropriate treatment during the acute stage of VKH disease, especially within the critical therapeutic window, often leads to progression to chronic disease. Chronic disease may manifest within several weeks to 9 months following the acute uveitis phase in 17–79% of patients [32, 33]. The chronic phase of VKH disease is characterized by a combination of choroidal atrophy and localized choroidal thickening, the latter resulting from new areas of inflammatory activity [34]. At this stage, active choroiditis typically resolves, leading to the development of a sunset glow fundus—a hallmark feature caused by depigmentation of the RPE and the underlying choroid, peripheral atrophic scars corresponding to regressed Dalen-Fuchs nodules, and pigmentary migration. Exudative retinal detachments often do not persist, although other signs of inflammation, such as "demarcation lines" indicating the extent of previous detachments, may remain present [35]. Chronic granulomatous or non-granulomatous anterior uveitis is a prominent feature of the chronic phase and typically presents with mutton-fat keratic precipitates (KPs), Koeppe nodules, Busacca nodules, and a marked anterior chamber inflammatory reaction. Managing the chronic phase of the disease requires extended therapy due to repeated flare-ups, most commonly involving the anterior segment.

Systemic manifestations poliosis, alopecia, and vitiligo, are more commonly observed extraocular findings at this stage [36].

The chronic form is frequently associated with complications [13]. Recurrent anterior segment inflammation and prolonged systemic corticosteroid therapy are recognized risk factors for complicated cataract, which represents one of the most frequent complications of VKH disease (10.5–42%) [37]. Another frequent complication is glaucoma, which develops in 6–45% of eyes [38]. Macular neovascularization occurs in fewer than 10% of cases, typically linked to fundus pigmentary alterations, more severe anterior chamber, and vitreous inflammation [39]. Macular edema may develop in approximately 5% of eyes, typically in association with prolonged inflammation during recurrent disease episodes, or in the presence of epiretinal membranes [40]. Neovascularization of the retina and optic nerve may occur, leading to recurrent and clinically significant vitreous hemorrhages [41]. Subretinal fibrosis, though uncommon, is a more serious and potentially vision-threatening complication in chronic VKH [15].

3. Diagnostic criteria

The diagnosis of VKH syndrome is primarily established through clinical findings and by ruling out other potential diseases [10]. The mandatory diagnostic criteria mainly include the absence of any prior ocular trauma or intraocular surgery before the onset of uveitis, bilateral ocular involvement, and the exclusion of other possible causes of uveitis based on clinical and laboratory evaluations [2].

Several diagnostic criteria have been established for the diagnosis of VHK disease. In 1978, the American Uveitis Society established the following diagnostic criteria for VKH disease, aiming to standardize clinical diagnosis: (1) the absence of any history of ocular trauma or surgery; and (2) the presence of at least three of the following four signs: (a) bilateral chronic iridocyclitis; (b) posterior uveitis, including exudative retinal detachment, forme fruste of exudative retinal detachment, disc hyperemia or edema, and a "sunsetglow" fundus; (c) neurologic signs, such as tinnitus, neck stiffness, cranial nerve abnormalities, central nervous system disorders, or cerebrospinal fluid pleocytosis; and (d) cutaneous manifestations, including alopecia, poliosis, or vitiligo [26]. In 2000, Read et al. [42] conducted a retrospective review of 71 patients with VKH disease, applying the then-existing diagnostic criteria. Their findings revealed that approximately half of the patients did not meet the criteria for diagnosis. They concluded that the criteria were not practical for diagnostic purposes, as they required chronic intraocular cellular inflammation or initial skin findings, both of which are rarely observed during the acute phase. Consequently, revised diagnostic criteria for VKH disease were proposed at the First International Workshop on Vogt-Koyanagi-Harada Disease in 2001, as summarized in **Table 1** [43].

An analysis based on the revised diagnostic criteria for VKH disease revealed that 12% of cases were classified as complete VKH, 71% as incomplete VKH, and 9% as probable VKH [44]. One contributing factor to the low proportion of cases being classified as complete VKH under the revised diagnostic criteria is the use of modern corticosteroid therapy, which can prevent the progression to late-stage disease.

1. No history of penetrating ocular trauma or surgery preceding the initial onset of uveitis
2. No clinical or laboratory evidence suggestive of other ocular disease entities
3. Bilateral ocular involvement (A or B must be met, depending on the stage of disease when the patient is examined):
   a. *Early manifestations of disease:*
      i. Evidence of diffuse choroiditis (with or without anterior uveitis, vitreous inflammatory reaction, or optic disc hyperemia), which may manifest as one of the following:
         a. *Focal areas of subretinal fluid, or*
         b. *Bullous exudative retinal detachments*
      ii. With equivocal fundus findings, both of the following must be present as well:
         a. *Focal areas of delay in choroidal perfusion, multifocal areas of pinpoint leakage, large placoid areas of hyperfluorescence, pooling within subretinal fluid, and optic nerve staining (listed in order of sequential appearance) by fluorescein angiography and*
         b. *Diffuse choroidal thickening, without evidence of posterior scleritis by ultrasonography*
   a. *Late manifestations of disease:*
      i. History suggestive of prior presence of early findings noted in 3A and either (II) or (III) below, or multiple signs from (III) below:
      ii. Ocular depigmentation: either
         a. *Sunset glow fundus or*
         b. *Sugiura's sign*
      iii. Other ocular signs, including
         a. *Nummular chorioretinal depigmented scars, or*
         b. *Retinal pigment epithelium clumping and/or migration, or*
         c. *Recurrent or chronic anterior uveitis*
4. Neurological/auditory findings (may resolve by time of evaluation):
   a. *Meningismus (malaise, fever, headache, nausea, abdominal pain, stiffness of the neck and back, or a combination of these factors); note that headache alone is not sufficient to meet the definition of meningismus.*
   b. *Tinnitus*
   c. *Cerebrospinal fluid pleocytosis*

5. Integumentary findings (not preceding the onset of central nervous system or ocular disease):
    a. *Alopecia, or*
    b. *Poliosis, or*
    c. *Vitiligo*

Complete Vogt-Koyanagi-Harada disease: criteria 1–5 must be present
Incomplete Vogt-Koyanagi-Harada disease: criteria 1–3 and either 4 or 5 must be present
Probable Vogt-Koyanagi-Harada disease (isolated ocular disease): criteria 1–3 must be present.

Table 1.
Revised criteria for diagnosis of Vogt-Koyanagi-Harada disease.

In 2021, the Standardization of Uveitis Nomenclature (SUN) Working Group, an international collaboration tasked with developing formal classification criteria for 25 common uveitic diseases, introduced distinct criteria that separately specify the early and late stages of VKH disease (**Tables 2** and **3**) [45].

In 2022, Herbort et al. [15] critically reviewed emerging concepts and novel diagnostic approaches for VKH disease, highlighting several key updates for early diagnosis: (1) a fundamental distinction between acute initial-onset and chronic forms of the disease; (2) the incorporation of advanced imaging modalities for precise assessment of choroidal inflammation; (3) the endorsement of simplified and more reliable diagnostic criteria for acute initial-onset VKH, centered on the essential finding of diffuse choroiditis, as identified by indocyanine green angiography (ICGA) and/or enhanced depth imaging optical coherence tomography (EDI-OCT); and (4) the emphasis on optimizing treatment through early, aggressive, and sustained administration of corticosteroids combined with

Criteria (Diagnosis requires #1 or #2 AND #3)

1. Evidence of Harada disease
    a. Serous (exudative) retinal detachment AND (b. and/or c.)
    b. Multiloculated appearance on fluorescein angiogram OR
    c. Septae on optical coherence tomogram

OR

2. Panuveitis[a] with ≥2 of the following neurologic symptoms or signs[b]
    a. Headache OR
    b. Tinnitus OR
    c. Dysacusis OR
    d. Meningismus OR
    e. Cerebrospinal fluid pleocytosis

AND

3. No history of penetrating ocular trauma or vitreoretinal surgery before disease onset

Exclusions

1. Positive serology for syphilis using a treponemal test
2. Evidence for sarcoidosis (either bilateral hilar adenopathy on chest imaging or tissue biopsy demonstrating noncaseating granulomata)

[a]*Uveitis should have evidence of choroidal involvement on clinical examination, fluorescein angiography, indocyanine green angiography, or optical coherence tomography, including enhanced depth imaging of the choroid.*
[b]*Onset of neurologic symptoms and signs and onset of the uveitis should occur within 4 weeks of each other.*

Table 2.
Classification criteria for early-stage Vogt-Koyanagi-Harada disease.

Criteria
1. History of early-stage Vogt-Koyanagi-Harada disease
AND (#2 and/or #3)
2. Sunset glow fundus
OR
3. Uveitis* AND ≥ 1 of the following cutaneous findings
a. Vitiligo OR
b. Poliosis OR
c. Alopecia
Exclusions
1. Positive serology for syphilis using a treponemal test
2. Evidence for sarcoidosis (either bilateral hilar adenopathy on chest imaging or tissue biopsy demonstrating noncaseating granulomata)

Uveitis may be:
1) Chronic anterior uveitis;
2) Anterior and intermediate uveitis; or
3) Panuveitis with multifocal choroiditis (Dalen-Fuchs-like nodules)

Table 3.
Classification criteria for late-stage Vogt-Koyanagi-Harada disease.

1. No ocular trauma or surgery preceding disease onset[a]
2. Bilateral involvement (verified with ICGA and/or EDI-OCT)[a]
3. Exclusion of other infectious, inflammatory, or masquerading entities, particularly other stromal choroiditis entities (e.g., tuberculosis, sarcoidosis, or syphilis)[a]
4. Diffuse choroiditis, evidenced by ICGA and/or EDI-OCT[a]
5. Signs and symptoms have persisted for less than 4 weeks[a]
6. Absence of clinical findings compatible with chronic disease (i.e., sunset glow fundus or integumentary signs, like vitiligo, alopecia, or poliosis)[a]
7. Exudative retinal detachment (evidenced by pooling and pinpoint leakage on FA and ICGA) (a very helpful criterion when present)
8. Disc hyperfluorescence (a helpful criterion)
9. Neurological/auditory findings (meningismus, tinnitus, acute hearing loss) (a helpful criterion)

FA, fluorescein angiography; ICGA, indocyanine green angiography; EDI-OCT, enhanced depth imaging optical coherence tomography.[a]Essential required criteria.

Table 4.
The proposed new diagnostic criteria for initial-onset Vogt-Koyanagi-Harada disease.

nonsteroidal immunosuppressive agents, along with vigilant monitoring of subclinical choroidal inflammation during follow-up (**Table 4**).

4. Imaging methods

4.1 Optical coherence tomography

Optical coherence tomography (OCT) has emerged as an indispensable imaging modality in the assessment of VKH disease, enabling detailed visualization of retinal and choroidal structures that are often difficult to evaluate through the conventional clinical examination alone [14, 46]. In the acute phase, OCT commonly reveals exudative retinal detachments, often accompanied by subretinal septa—structures believed to be composed of inflammatory materials [47]. These septa have been hypothesized to result either from inflammatory deposits [48] or from a separation between the inner and outer segments of photoreceptors combined with fibrin accumulation [49]. A significant proportion of eyes in the acute stage exhibit intraretinal and subretinal fluid accumulation on OCT. Fluid in the outer retinal layers, associated with severe dye leakage from RPE, was reported in 40% of eyes with VKH disease [50]. Additionally, features such as undulations, previously attributed to the choroid, have been clarified through OCT to actually represent undulations of the RPE itself [51]. The subretinal fluid correlates with initial visual acuity in eyes with VKH disease. However, this parameter does not predict time to resolution or final visual outcome. The presence of choroidal folds and multifocal retinal detachments is reported to be associated with baseline visual acuity, but it does not correlate with visual outcomes or subretinal fluid resolution (**Figure 2**) [52].

Enhanced depth imaging (EDI) OCT, an advanced imaging technique capable of detecting choroidal changes, has enabled detailed evaluation of choroidal thickening in acute VKH disease [14]. The choroid is significantly thicker in the acute stage of VKH disease, compared to convalescent-stage patients and healthy eyes [53, 54]. A rapid decrease in choroidal thickness following corticosteroid treatment has also been reported in these eyes [55]. Changes in choroidal thickness not only reflect treatment

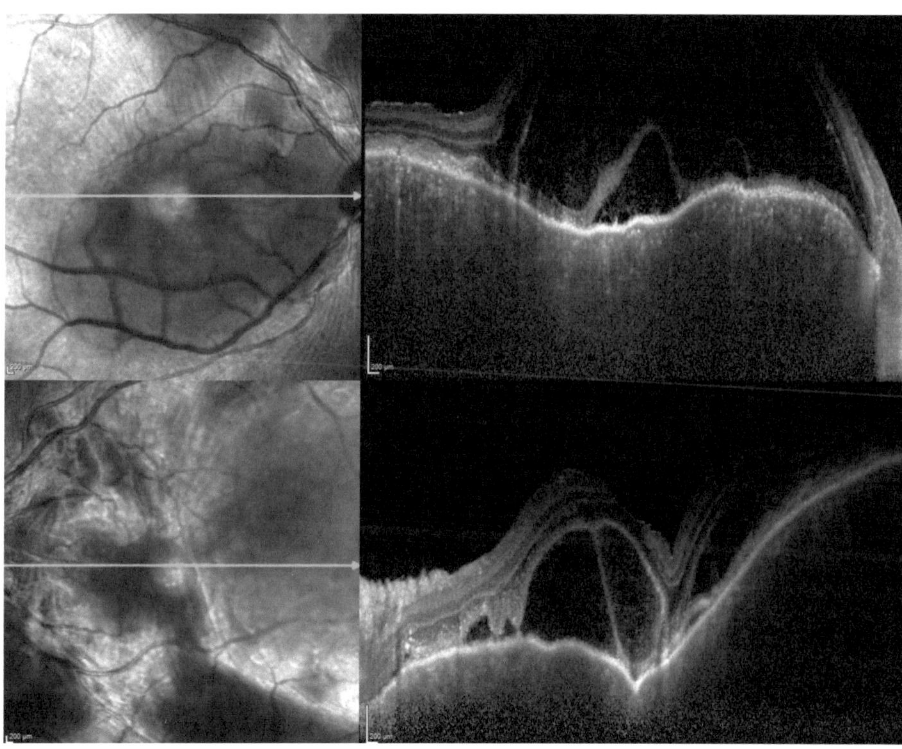

Figure 2.
Spectral-domain optical coherence tomography (OCT) sections demonstrating bilateral exudative retinal detachments with subretinal septa formation, markedly thickened choroid, bacillary layer detachment, and chorioretinal undulations in a patient with early-stage Vogt-Koyanagi-Harada disease (Courtesy of Ali Osman Saatci, MD).

efficacy but may also serve as indicators of disease recurrence. For instance, recurrence can be accompanied by an increase in choroidal thickness or the reappearance of choroidal folds [56]. In contrast, the convalescent phase and chronic stages of VKH—particularly in eyes exhibiting the characteristic sunset glow fundus—are associated with choroidal thinning [14]. Histopathological studies have corroborated these findings, revealing choroidal melanocyte loss and choroidal atrophy during the convalescent and chronic recurrent stages of VKH. Additionally, loss of the choriocapillaris has been noted in the convalescent phase, further contributing to choroidal thinning. The reductions in choroidal thickness observed on OCT likely reflect these histological changes [46].

4.2 Fundus autofluorescence

Fundus autofluorescence (FAF), which primarily visualizes lipofuscin accumulation within the RPE, has emerged as a valuable imaging modality in the assessment of VKH disease. It facilitates the detection of RPE abnormalities that may not be apparent on clinical examination and the extent of posterior segment involvement with widefield imaging [57]. In the acute phase of VKH, FAF typically demonstrates a diffusely increased autofluorescent signal, often accompanied by areas of signal blockage corresponding to exudative retinal detachments observed at the onset of symptoms. These abnormal signals usually resolve following high-dose intravenous corticosteroid therapy. However, in patients who present later in the disease course, FAF often reveals a mottled pattern of hyperautofluorescence interspersed with hypoautofluorescent zones, particularly in areas previously affected by subretinal fluid (**Figure 3**) [58].

4.3 Fluorescein angiography

Advancements in imaging technology have significantly enhanced the ability to visualize and comprehend the pathophysiological mechanisms involved in

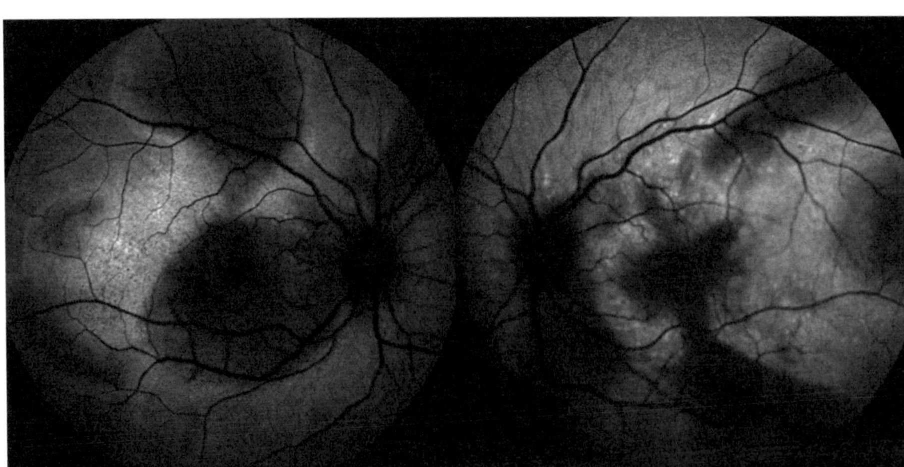

Figure 3.
Fundus autofluorescence imaging demonstrating bilateral patchy hypoautofluorescent areas corresponding to exudative retinal detachments with surrounding hyperautofluorescent borders, consistent with retinal pigment epithelium alterations in the early stage of Vogt-Koyanagi-Harada disease (Courtesy of Ali Osman Saatci, MD).

VKH-affected eyes. Among these modalities, FA remains one of the earliest and most extensively utilized techniques [1]. It plays a pivotal role in evaluating retinal and choroidal alterations across the disease course.

In the acute phase of VKH disease, FA findings include optic disc hyperfluorescence (94.4%), alongside disseminated spotted choroidal hyperfluorescence and delayed choroidal filling (83.3%). During the chronic uveitic stage, the most common findings are reported as spotted hyperfluorescence and hypofluorescence (72.7%), as well as optic disc hyperfluorescence (72.7%). Retinal vascular hyperfluorescence is less common, present in 18.2% of patients. In the convalescent phase, FA often demonstrates spotted hyper- and hypofluorescence (73.3%), blockage of choroidal fluorescence secondary to RPE migration (56.7%), and dot-like hyperfluorescence in the equatorial retina (43.3%). These equatorial findings frequently correlate with clinically visible nummular white scars, a hallmark of the healing phase of VKH [24].

Chee et al. [59] provided additional insight by describing early pinpoint peripapillary hyperfluorescence on FA in patients imaged within 14 days of symptom onset. This "hyperacute" finding was associated with a favorable prognosis and disease resolution. In contrast, patients lacking this angiographic sign required more prolonged and aggressive immunosuppressive therapy, likely due to delayed initiation of treatment. Thus, early peripapillary leakage on FA may serve as a valuable prognostic marker for disease staging and therapeutic planning (**Figure 4**) [59].

4.4 Indocyanine green angiography

Indocyanine green angiography is a useful imaging modality for visualizing chorioretinal involvement in VKH disease [60]. It offers complementary insights into VKH disease by enabling deeper imaging of the choroidal vasculature. It is particularly useful for detecting early choroidal vasculopathy, characterized by fuzzy, indistinct vessels and diffuse choroidal hyperfluorescence, indicative of underlying inflammatory processes [61].

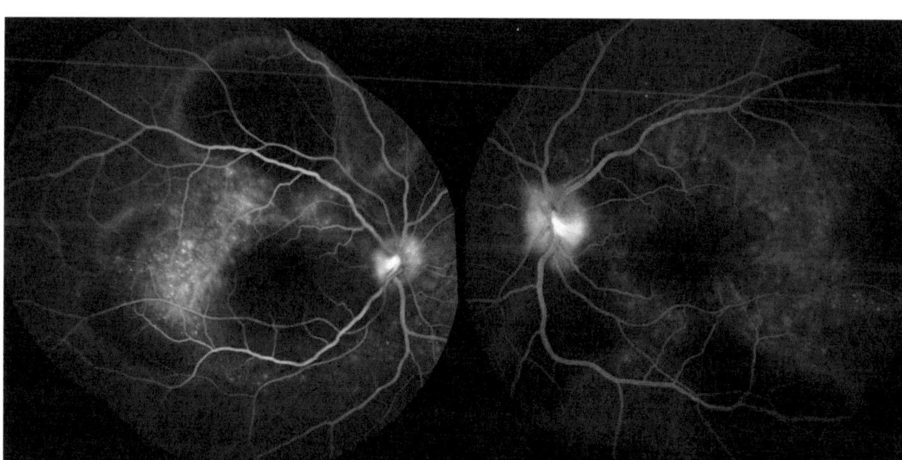

Figure 4.
Late-phase fundus fluorescein angiography depicting bilateral multiple punctate hyperfluorescent spots with pooling and staining, along with optic disc leakage in early-stage Vogt-Koyanagi-Harada disease (Courtesy of Ali Osman Saatci, MD).

Recent advances in OCT technology, particularly those allowing precise measurement of choroidal thickness, may begin to provide similarly valuable diagnostic and monitoring capabilities. However, ICGA remains the gold standard for directly visualizing inflammatory changes within the choroidal stroma, especially during subclinical or recurrent disease phases. Multiple studies have shown that ICGA is highly sensitive in diagnosing initial-onset VKH, with some reporting 100% sensitivity and others noting sensitivities greater than 90% [62–64].

Typical ICGA findings in VKH include hyperfluorescent areas, hypofluorescent dark spots, and optic disc hyperfluorescence—features more readily visualized in severe or active disease. These findings reflect granulomatous choroiditis and persistent stromal inflammation, often undetectable on clinical examination or FA [65]. Importantly, ICGA can also identify subclinical inflammation, particularly during corticosteroid tapering or in suspected relapses [14]. The ability to detect occult disease activity with ICGA can inform treatment adjustments, potentially necessitating prolonged immunosuppression to prevent chronic complications such as the sunset glow fundus. Studies showed the clinical utility of ICGA in revealing persistent choroidal inflammation in VKH and other granulomatous diseases, such as ocular sarcoidosis, tuberculosis, and birdshot chorioretinopathy [61].

Choroidal venous overload is another finding defined in patients with VKH disease with the help of angiographic techniques. In a retrospective study by Noh et al. [66], 52 eyes with VKH disease and 24 control eyes underwent multimodal imaging, including FA and ICGA. The findings revealed that angiographic signs of choroidal venous overload, such as intervortex venous anastomosis, were present in eyes with VKH disease.

In the chronic phase, FAF findings become more variable and may include both increased and decreased autofluorescence patterns. Decreased autofluorescence is typically indicative of RPE atrophy or outer retinal involvement and is commonly seen in peripapillary atrophy and nummular chorioretinal scars. Conversely, areas of increased autofluorescence may reflect the presence of cystoid macular edema, subretinal fibrosis, or zones of RPE proliferation [67].

4.5 Ultrasonography

While the diagnosis of VKH disease is predominantly clinical, there are instances in which direct visualization of the posterior segment is impeded. Media opacities, such as dense vitritis, posterior synechiae, or cataract, can obscure the view, complicating posterior segment evaluation. In such scenarios, B-scan ultrasonography serves as a valuable diagnostic adjunct. Typical ultrasonographic findings consistent with VKH include: (1) diffuse, low to medium reflective thickening of the choroid posteriorly; (2) serous retinal detachment located inferiorly or in the posterior pole; (3) mild vitreous opacities with no posterior vitreous detachment; and (4) thickening of the sclera and/or episclera posteriorly. Moreover, ultrasonography proves useful in monitoring treatment response, as progressive resolution of these findings often parallels clinical improvement with corticosteroid and immunosuppressive therapy [14].

An unusual but clinically significant presentation of VKH involves secondary angle-closure glaucoma. Such presentations may be erroneously interpreted as acute angle-closure glaucoma, potentially leading to inappropriate management [68]. Ultrasound biomicroscopy can assist clinicians in such cases by revealing a shallow anterior chamber, narrow anterior chamber angles, detachment of the ciliary body, and peripheral choroidal effusions [14, 68].

4.6 Optical coherence tomography angiography

Optical coherence tomography angiography is a noninvasive imaging tool that provides high-resolution, three-dimensional maps of chorioretinal circulation without the need for dye injections, allowing for quantitative assessment of retinal and choroidal vascular structures [69]. It can detect perfusion deficits in both the superficial and deep capillary plexuses, a feature that fluorescein angiography cannot achieve [70]. It is widely used to study retinal microvascular changes in uveitis, including VKH disease.

Research on OCT angiography in VKH disease has shown contradictory results. Some studies indicate that choroidal capillary vascular density is higher in recovering VKH patients compared to controls [71, 72], while others report the opposite [73, 74]. Additionally, variations in the foveal avascular zone (FAZ) size have been observed. Some studies showed a larger FAZ in remission-phase VKH disease [71, 75], while others report a smaller FAZ in recovery-phase patients [72]. The contradictory findings among studies may be attributed to differences in imaging devices, image analysis protocols, or the disease stage at the time of evaluation. A recent meta-analysis found that both the superficial capillary plexus and deep capillary plexus vessel densities in the macula were lower in VKH patients during the active phase compared to those in remission and normal individuals. Additionally, choriocapillary vascular density was reduced during the active phase in comparison to remission, and patients in remission had a larger FAZ than normal individuals [76].

5. Differential diagnosis

The differential diagnosis of VKH disease is broad and necessitates a structured and methodical approach. The first critical step is to assess for any history of ocular trauma. If such a history is present, sympathetic ophthalmia should be prominently considered. In the absence of trauma, the differential should expand to include infectious etiologies, masquerade syndromes, and noninfectious inflammatory conditions (**Table 5**).

Sympathetic ophthalmia closely resembles VKH disease in both clinical and histopathological features. However, it typically occurs in the setting of prior ocular trauma or surgery, which is absent in VKH. A history of penetrating injury and a unilateral onset that evolves into bilateral disease are distinguishing clues favoring sympathetic ophthalmia [77].

Sarcoidosis can present with bilateral uveitis and choroidal granulomas, mimicking VKH. However, the presence of systemic findings, such as bilateral hilar lymphadenopathy on chest imaging and noncaseating granulomas on biopsy, is characteristic of sarcoidosis. Moreover, periphlebitis and "candle-wax drippings" on fundus examination are more typical of sarcoidosis than VKH [78].

Posterior scleritis can cause exudative retinal detachment and choroidal thickening, features also seen in VKH. However, patients with posterior scleritis often experience significant ocular pain, and B-mode ultrasonography typically reveals a characteristic "T-sign" due to fluid in Tenon's capsule, which is absent in VKH [79].

Intraocular lymphoma may masquerade as chronic posterior uveitis and should be suspected in older patients with an atypical presentation, poor response to corticosteroids, or vitritis with subretinal infiltrates. Diagnostic confirmation often requires vitreous biopsy and cytologic evaluation [14].

1. **History of trauma**
Sympathetic ophthalmia
2. **Infections**
Tuberculosis
Syphilis
Other bacterial infections (Lyme, cat-scratch, etc.)
Fungal infections
3. **Malignancies**
Systemic lymphoma or leukemia
Intraocular lymphoma
Diffuse uveal lymphoid hyperplasia
Bilateral diffuse uveal melanocytic hyperplasia
Monoclonal gammopathies
Metastatic carcinoma
4. **Inflammatory conditions**
Bilateral posterior scleritis
Acute posterior multifocal placoid pigment epitheliopathy
Sarcoidosis
Multiple evanescent white dot syndrome
Lupus choroidopathy
5. **Other entities**
Eclampsia
Malignant hypertension
Serum calcium abnormalities
Central serous chorioretinopathy
Uveal effusion syndrome

Table 5.
Differential diagnosis of Vogt-Koyanagi-Harada disease.

6. Treatment options

The key principle in treating VKH disease is to manage the initial eye inflammation during the acute posterior uveitic phase with early and strong immunosuppressive therapy. This may shorten the disease duration, lower the risk of becoming chronic, and reduce the risk of systemic symptoms [15].

6.1 Corticosteroids

Early and prompt administration of high-dose systemic corticosteroids, with a slow tapering schedule extending over three to six months, remains the gold standard treatment approach for VKH disease [10, 79]. A typical treatment regimen includes a 3-day course of intravenous methylprednisolone (500–1000 mg/day), followed by high-dose oral prednisone (1 mg/kg) for a duration of 4–6 weeks [15]. Despite its therapeutic benefits, systemic corticosteroid therapy carries multiple side effects—such as cataracts, ocular hypertension, gastrointestinal issues, hyperglycemia, osteoporosis, femoral head osteonecrosis, and insomnia—that often limit its long-term use [8].

In patients presenting with marked serous retinal detachment, intravitreal and/or posterior subtenon's injection of corticosteroids may serve as an effective adjunct to systemic corticosteroid therapy. This local corticosteroid delivery can enhance control of posterior segment inflammation, particularly in the early stages of the disease. Additionally, in cases with significant anterior chamber inflammation, topical corticosteroid eye drops can be beneficial in managing anterior segment involvement [7].

Although systemic corticosteroid therapy is considered the cornerstone of initial treatment in early-onset VKH disease, its prompt administration does not consistently prevent progression to the chronic recurrent stage in a substantial proportion of patients [33, 80]. Chee et al. [81] found that approximately one-third of patients who received corticosteroid therapy within 2 weeks of symptom onset progressed to chronic recurrent disease. Keino et al. [82] also demonstrated that 17.5% of patients developed chronic ocular inflammation despite prompt initiation of high-dose corticosteroids at the initial onset of VKH. These findings underscore the critical need for long-term immunosuppressive therapy in patients with VKH disease to achieve sustained disease control and prevent chronic recurrence.

6.2 Immunosuppressive agents

In addition to corticosteroids, immunosuppressive agents, such as mycophenolate mofetil, methotrexate, azathioprine, cyclosporine A, and alkylating agents, have been successfully employed in the management of VKH disease. The American Uveitis Society and the International Uveitis Study Group recommend the use of such immunosuppressive agents as essential components of the treatment of VKH disease [14, 83]. A careful balance is required between initiating prompt corticosteroid treatment and implementing timely immunosuppressive therapy to optimize long-term disease control and minimize recurrences.

Mycophenolate mofetil has demonstrated efficacy as a corticosteroid-sparing agent in uncontrolled studies on noninfectious uveitis. Evidence from the literature suggests that mycophenolate mofetil, whether used in combination with systemic corticosteroids or other immunosuppressive agents, is associated with improved visual outcomes and a reduced risk of progression to chronic disease compared to corticosteroid monotherapy in patients with acute VKH disease [84, 85]. Its immunosuppressive activity is mediated through the reversible inhibition of inosine-5′-monophosphate dehydrogenase, a key enzyme in the *de novo* purine synthesis pathway, thereby suppressing lymphocyte proliferation. This ultimately inhibits the proliferation of both T and B lymphocytes, thereby attenuating the immune-mediated inflammatory response [86]. Mycophenolate mofetil is usually given orally at a dose of 0.5–2 g/day or 10–30 mg/kg/day and may cause gastrointestinal side effects, such as nausea, vomiting, diarrhea, and loss of appetite. Additionally, it can lead to less common side effects, including liver and kidney toxicity, bone marrow suppression, and an elevated risk of infections and tumors. Regular monitoring is crucial to manage these risks [87].

Methotrexate is a folate analog that inhibits dihydrofolate reductase, thereby blocking the synthesis of tetrahydrofolate and disrupting nucleic acid and protein synthesis. Although more limited, existing studies suggest that methotrexate may also serve as an effective adjunct to corticosteroid therapy in the management of VKH-associated uveitis, contributing to inflammation control and potentially reducing the risk of disease chronicity [88, 89]. Methotrexate is associated with several common adverse effects, including bone marrow suppression, hepatotoxicity, pulmonary toxicity, gastrointestinal disturbances, alopecia, and dermatitis. To reduce the risk of hematologic and other complications, it is recommended to supplement treatment with folic acid (1 mg/day) or folinic acid, and to closely monitor blood counts and liver function throughout the course of therapy [90]. Recently, the First-Line Antimetabolites for Steroid-Sparing Treatment Uveitis Trial demonstrated that there was no significant difference in the efficacy of methotrexate compared to mycophenolate mofetil in achieving disease control in patients with VKH [91].

Azathioprine is an antimetabolite with cytostatic properties that target dividing cells [92]. Azathioprine, administered at a dose of 1–2.5 mg/kg/day, has been reported to be effective in controlling disease progression in VKH disease, particularly in patients who are nonresponsive or poorly responsive to corticosteroids, as well as in those who exhibit steroid intolerance [93]. Azathioprine typically takes 2–3 months to reach its full therapeutic effect. As a result, it is recommended to use corticosteroids concurrently during the initial phase of treatment to provide rapid and effective control of acute inflammatory episodes. Given its potential hematologic and hepatic toxicity, regular monitoring of complete blood counts and liver enzyme levels is crucial during azathioprine treatment (**Figure 5**) [90].

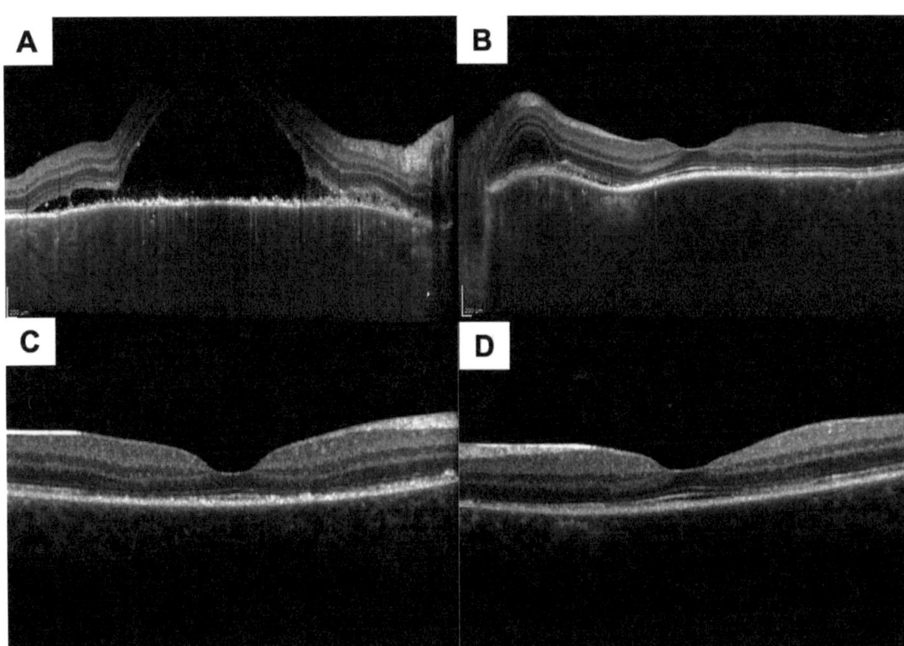

Figure 5.
Spectral-domain optical coherence tomography images of a 24-year-old female patient with Vogt-Koyanagi-Harada disease at admission, showing bilateral serous retinal detachment and subretinal septa, hyperreflective dots in the subretinal space, and markedly thickened choroid with mild undulation (A, right eye; and B, left eye). Follow-up images obtained 20 days after initiation of systemic corticosteroid and azathioprine therapy demonstrating complete resolution of subretinal fluid and restoration of normal foveal contour, while the choroid remains thickened (C, right eye; and D, left eye) (Courtesy of Ali Osman Saatci, MD).

Cyclosporine A, a T-lymphocyte inhibitor that inhibits calcineurin, administered at a dose of 2–5 mg/kg/day, is among the most widely used immunosuppressive agents in the management of VKH disease. Previous studies show that cyclosporine A is a better glucocorticoid-sparing agent as compared to azathioprine [94]. Cyclosporine A is associated with several side effects, the most notable being nephrotoxicity and hypertension, necessitating regular monitoring of serum creatinine levels and blood pressure. Common adverse effects also include gingival hyperplasia, hypertrichosis, acroparesthesias, and cholestatic hepatitis. Long-term use has been linked to an increased risk of lymphoproliferative disorders and malignant skin tumors, underscoring the need for careful surveillance during therapy [92].

6.3 Biological agents

Biologic agents represent a modern therapeutic approach for managing ocular inflammatory diseases. The American Uveitis Society expert panel issued guidelines recommending TNF blockers—specifically infliximab and adalimumab—as potential second-line immunomodulatory therapies for severe forms of uveitis, including posterior and diffuse uveitis [95].

Infliximab is a widely used immunomodulatory agent in the management of various immune-mediated diseases, including rheumatoid arthritis, psoriasis, Crohn's disease, ankylosing spondylitis, and sarcoidosis. It is a chimeric monoclonal immunoglobulin G (IgG) antibody composed of both murine and human components, specifically targeting TNF-α. Infliximab has demonstrated significant clinical efficacy, particularly in cases that were previously difficult to manage, underscoring the pivotal role of TNF-α in the pathogenesis of autoimmune disorders [96]. Infliximab is typically administered *via* intravenous infusion at doses ranging from 3 to 10 mg/kg, with higher doses up to 20 mg/kg also reported as effective and well-tolerated in certain cases with VKH disease [97].

Adalimumab, a biologic agent targeting TNF-α, is an approved treatment for noninfectious uveitis. Its efficacy and safety in patients with VKH disease have been demonstrated in phase 3 randomized controlled trials [98]. It is already widely used worldwide for diseases, such as rheumatoid arthritis and Crohn's disease and has shown outstanding therapeutic efficacy. The standard dosing regimen for adalimumab in the treatment of noninfectious uveitis is 40 mg every 2 weeks. The steroid-sparing effect of adalimumab in VKH disease has been well documented, with a mean reduction of 62.7% reported in the study by Shinagawa et al. [8]. Observational studies have also demonstrated that adalimumab is effective in achieving remission in certain patients with refractory VKH disease [99]. In a recent multicenter study, Nakai et al. [99] retrospectively examined 70 VKH patients who had received adalimumab treatment for over 6 months. They found that adalimumab was effective in achieving and maintaining remission of ocular inflammation in VKH patients who were resistant to conventional immunosuppressive therapies [99].

Despite their efficacy, anti-TNF agents are associated with notable adverse effects, including reactivation of latent infections (particularly tuberculosis), demyelinating diseases, exacerbation of congestive heart failure, lupus-like syndromes, and an increased risk of malignancies [100].

B cells, in conjunction with T lymphocytes, play a crucial role in the onset and progression of autoimmune diseases. Beyond producing autoantibodies, B cells can capture antigens through their B-cell receptors and contribute to autoimmunity by presenting autoantigens to pathogenic T cells. Although not routinely employed in the management of VKH disease, B-cell depletion therapy with the anti-CD20 monoclonal antibody rituximab is considered a viable treatment option for patients with refractory, chronic recurrent uveitis associated with VKH disease [15, 101, 102]. The most commonly reported adverse event associated with rituximab therapy is an infusion-related reaction [103].

7. Challenges in management

Despite significant advances in imaging techniques and therapeutic interventions, managing VKH disease continues to present considerable challenges. Early diagnosis of VKH disease presents a significant challenge, as prodromal symptoms are often nonspecific and can mimic other neurological or systemic disorders. Moreover, in the initial stages, the hallmark clinical features of VKH may not yet be fully evident, further complicating timely and accurate diagnosis.

While current monitoring tools have improved, they may still fail to reliably detect subclinical inflammation, leading to delayed identification of relapses. Additionally, high relapse rates persist, even with the early use of corticosteroids, highlighting the critical need for more effective long-term immunomodulatory strategies [13, 33]. The development of personalized management plans, tailored to the individual patient's response and disease progression, is essential to improving outcomes and minimizing the risk of recurrence.

8. Prognosis

The long-term visual prognosis in VKH disease is primarily influenced by early diagnosis, prompt initiation of high-dose corticosteroid therapy, and sustained immunosuppressive treatment. Aggressive and timely intervention can result in significantly improved visual outcomes. The initiation of high-dose corticosteroids within the first few weeks of disease onset is critical [14]. Prolonged corticosteroid therapy is often required to control inflammation effectively. Studies report final visual acuity in VKH patients ranging from 20/20 to 20/50, emphasizing the potential for recovery with appropriate management [104].

Advancements in imaging techniques, including ICGA and OCT, play a crucial role in detecting subclinical disease and assessing treatment efficacy. These imaging modalities allow for the identification of choroidal inflammation and the monitoring of choroidal thickness, providing valuable insights into disease progression and treatment response. The use of these advanced imaging techniques may extend the duration of treatment and help reduce the risk of complications, such as sunset glow fundus and choroidal thinning [57].

The extent of choroidal involvement, persistence of inflammation, and effective control of subclinical choroidal inflammation, as indicated by decreasing choroidal thickness on OCT, are important determinants of long-term prognosis. The presence of secondary complications, such as cataract, glaucoma, or macular neovascularization, can negatively impact the final visual acuity and should be managed promptly [14].

9. New developments and future directions

Recent advances in both imaging and therapeutic modalities have opened new avenues for the diagnosis, monitoring, and management of VKH disease. One

DOI: http://dx.doi.org/10.5772/intechopen.1010862

such advancement is the application of widefield OCT angiography. It enables the noninvasive identification of flow voids at the level of superficial choroidal vessels during the acute phase of VKH disease. Given its ability to detect subtle vascular abnormalities, widefield OCT angiography may serve as a valuable adjunct in the diagnosis, monitoring of disease activity, and assessment of therapeutic response in VKH disease [105].

From a therapeutic standpoint, there is growing interest in targeted immunomodulatory therapies, particularly IL-6 inhibitors and Janus kinase (JAK) inhibitors, which have demonstrated promise in other autoimmune and inflammatory conditions. IL-6 inhibitors, such as tocilizumab, have emerged as promising therapeutic options for patients with refractory VKH disease or who develop complications such as cystoid macular edema [106]. JAK inhibitors, including agents such as tofacitinib and baricitinib, are currently under investigation for their capacity to modulate multiple cytokine signaling pathways simultaneously. This broader mechanism of action offers potential for effective control of both ocular and systemic inflammation. A variety of JAK inhibitors have been developed or are in development for use in refractory cases and for the management of autoimmune diseases, such as rheumatoid arthritis, psoriatic arthritis, ulcerative colitis, and ankylosing spondylitis. In the context of autoimmune-mediated noninfectious uveitis, JAK inhibitors may represent a promising future therapeutic option for the management of VKH disease, particularly in patients who are unresponsive to conventional immunosuppressive therapy [107].

The integration of artificial intelligence (AI) tools into clinical practice represents a transformative development in the early detection and management of numerous disorders. AI-driven image analysis algorithms applied to OCT, fundus photography, and angiographic data can assist clinicians in identifying early signs of VKH, even prior to the manifestation of overt clinical symptoms. The machine learning component of artificial intelligence was instrumental in the development of the SUN criteria for the classification of Vogt-Koyanagi-Harada disease, highlighting the growing role of AI-based technologies in refining diagnostic frameworks [45]. These technologies may also enable risk stratification, automated monitoring of disease progression, and personalized treatment planning, thus enhancing overall patient outcomes.

10. Conclusion

Vogt-Koyanagi-Harada disease remains a complex, multisystem autoimmune condition with variable clinical presentation and significant potential for long-term visual impairment if not promptly recognized and aggressively treated. Recent advances in multimodal imaging, especially OCT and ICGA, have enhanced our ability to diagnose, monitor, and manage VKH disease with greater precision. Modern therapeutic strategies increasingly emphasize early, sustained immunosuppression beyond corticosteroids to reduce recurrence and prevent chronic complications. As the understanding of the disease's immunopathogenesis and clinical phenotypes continues to evolve, incorporating updated diagnostic frameworks and individualized treatment regimens will be essential in optimizing patient outcomes.

Conflict of interest

The author declares no conflict of interest.

Author details

Mustafa Kayabaşı
Department of Ophthalmology, Muş State Hospital, Muş, Turkey

*Address all correspondence to: mkayabasi94@gmail.com

References

[1] Burkholder BM. Vogt-Koyanagi-Harada disease. Current Opinion in Ophthalmology. 2015;**26**(6):506-511

[2] Austin D, Moore JS, Gangaputra S. Vogt-Koyanagi-Harada syndrome: A rare cause of panuveitis presenting as unilateral loss of visual acuity. Journal of Clinical Rheumatology. 2021;**27**(8s):S838-S8s9

[3] Vogt A. Fruhzeitiges Ergrauen der Zilien und Bemerkungen uber den sogenannten plotzlichen Eintritt dieser Veranderung. Klinische Monatsblätter für Augenheilkunde. 1906;**44**:228-242

[4] Koyanagi Y. Dysacousia, Alopecia und Poliosis bei schwere Uveitis nicht traumatischen Ursprunges. Klinische Monatsblätter für Augenheilkunde. 1929;**82**:194-211

[5] Jaffe NS. Syndrome of Vogt-Koyanagi*. American Journal of Ophthalmology. 1950;**33**(4):571-576

[6] Harada E. Acute diffuse choroiditis. Acta of the Japanese Ophthalmological Society. 1926;**30**:356-378

[7] Yang P, Ye Z. Vogt–Koyanagi–Harada disease. In: Yu HG, editor. Inflammatory and Infectious Ocular Disorders. Singapore: Springer Singapore; 2020. pp. 67-75

[8] Shinagawa M, Namba K, Mizuuchi K, Iwata D, Hase K, Suzuki K, et al. The steroid-sparing effect of adalimumab in the treatment for the recurrent phase of Vogt-Koyanagi-Harada disease. Ocular Immunology and Inflammation. 2023;**31**(3):501-505

[9] Pan D, Hirose T. Vogt-Koyanagi-Harada syndrome: Review of clinical features. Seminars in Ophthalmology. 2011;**26**(4-5):312-315

[10] Guayacán CL, Galindo-Mendez B, de-la-Torre A. Vogt-Koyanagi-Harada syndrome in a group of patients in two ophthalmology referral centers in Bogotá, Colombia. Ocular Immunology and Inflammation. 2018;**26**(7):1123-1127

[11] Al Hemidan AI, Tabbara KF, Althomali T. Vogt-Koyanagi-Harada associated with diabetes mellitus and celiac disease in a 3-year-old girl. European Journal of Ophthalmology. 2006;**16**(1):173-177

[12] Sugita S, Takase H, Kawaguchi T, Taguchi C, Mochizuki M. Cross-reaction between tyrosinase peptides and cytomegalovirus antigen by T cells from patients with Vogt-Koyanagi-Harada disease. International Ophthalmology. 2007;**27**(2-3):87-95

[13] Du L, Kijlstra A, Yang P. Vogt-Koyanagi-Harada disease: Novel insights into pathophysiology, diagnosis and treatment. Progress in Retinal and Eye Research. 2016;**52**:84-111

[14] O'Keefe GA, Rao NA. Vogt-Koyanagi-Harada disease. Survey of Ophthalmology. 2017;**62**(1):1-25

[15] Herbort CP Jr, Tugal-Tutkun I, Abu-El-Asrar A, Gupta A, Takeuchi M, Fardeau C, et al. Precise, simplified diagnostic criteria and optimised management of initial-onset Vogt-Koyanagi-Harada disease: An updated review. Eye (London, England). 2022;**36**(1):29-43

[16] Moorthy RS, Rajeev B, Smith RE, Rao NA. Incidence and management of cataracts in Vogt-Koyanagi-Harada

syndrome. American Journal of Ophthalmology. 1994;**118**(2):197-204

[17] Yang P, Ren Y, Li B, Fang W, Meng Q, Kijlstra A. Clinical characteristics of Vogt-Koyanagi-Harada syndrome in Chinese patients. Ophthalmology. 2007;**114**(3):606-614

[18] Khairallah AS. Headache as an initial manifestation of Vogt-Koyanagi-Harada disease. Saudi Journal of Ophthalmology. 2014;**28**(3):239-242

[19] Nussenblatt RB, Whitcup SM. Uveitis: Fundamentals and Clinical Practice. 4th ed. St. Louis, Mo: Mosby/Elsevier; 2010

[20] Kamondi A, Szegedi A, Papp A, Seres A, Szirmai I. Vogt-Koyanagi-Harada disease presenting initially as aseptic meningoencephalitis. European Journal of Neurology. 2000;**7**(6):719-722

[21] Rajendram R, Evans M, Khurana RN, Tsai JH, Rao NA. Vogt-Koyanagi-Harada disease presenting as optic neuritis. International Ophthalmology. 2007;**27**(2-3):217-220

[22] Fardeau C, Tran TH, Gharbi B, Cassoux N, Bodaghi B, LeHoang P. Retinal fluorescein and indocyanine green angiography and optical coherence tomography in successive stages of Vogt-Koyanagi-Harada disease. International Ophthalmology. 2007;**27**(2-3):163-172

[23] Ohno S, Minakawa R, Matsuda H. Clinical studies of Vogt-Koyanagi-Harada's disease. Japanese Journal of Ophthalmology. 1988;**32**(3):334-343

[24] Arellanes-Garcia L, Hernandez-Barrios M, Fromow-Guerra J, Cervantes-Fanning P. Fluorescein fundus angiographic findings in Vogt-Koyanagi-Harada syndrome. International Ophthalmology. 2007;**27**(2-3):155-161

[25] Oellers P, Jaffe GJ, Proia AD. Clinical-pathological correlation of Vogt-Koyanagi-Harada disease. JAMA Ophthalmology. 2016;**134**(3):343-345

[26] Alexander LJ. Retina, 5th ed. Optometry and Vision Science. 2013;**90**(12):1827-1837

[27] El-Asrar AMA, Berghmans N, Al-Obeidan SA, Gikandi PW, Opdenakker G, Van Damme J, et al. Differential CXC and CX3C chemokine expression profiles in aqueous humor of patients with specific endogenous uveitic entities. Investigative Ophthalmology & Visual Science. 2018;**59**(6):2222-2228

[28] Kimura R, Sakai M, Okabe H. Transient shallow anterior chamber as initial symptom in Harada's syndrome. Archives of Ophthalmology. 1981;**99**(9):1604-1606

[29] Mantovani A, Resta A, Herbort CP, Abu El Asrar A, Kawaguchi T, Mochizuki M, et al. Work-up, diagnosis and management of acute Vogt-Koyanagi-Harada disease: A case of acute myopization with granulomatous uveitis. International Ophthalmology. 2007;**27**(2-3):105-115

[30] Kimura R, Kasai M, Shoji K, Kanno C. Swollen ciliary processes as an initial symptom in Vogt-Koyanagi-Harada syndrome. American Journal of Ophthalmology. 1983;**95**(3):402-403

[31] Tan JJ, Rao NA. Vogt-Koyanagi-Harada disease and sympathetic ophthalmia. In: Posterior Uveitis: Advances in Imaging and Treatment. Cleveland, OH, USA: Springer; 2019. pp. 39-56

[32] Urzua CA, Herbort C Jr, Valenzuela RA, Abu El-Asrar AM, Arellanes-Garcia L, Schlaen A, et al. Initial-onset acute and chronic recurrent

stages are two distinctive courses of Vogt-Koyanagi-Harada disease. Journal of Ophthalmic Inflammation and Infection. 2020;**10**(1):23

[33] Sakata VM, da Silva FT, Hirata CE, Marin ML, Rodrigues H, Kalil J, et al. High rate of clinical recurrence in patients with Vogt-Koyanagi-Harada disease treated with early high-dose corticosteroids. Graefe's Archive for Clinical and Experimental Ophthalmology. 2015;**253**(5):785-790

[34] Attia S, Khochtali S, Kahloun R, Zaouali S, Khairallah M. Vogt–Koyanagi–Harada disease. Expert Review of Ophthalmology. 2012;**7**(6):565-585

[35] da Silva FT, Hirata CE, Sakata VM, Olivalves E, Preti R, Pimentel SL, et al. Indocyanine green angiography findings in patients with long-standing Vogt-Koyanagi-Harada disease: A cross-sectional study. BMC Ophthalmology. 2012;**12**:40

[36] Noguchi Y, Nishio A, Takase H, Miyanaga M, Takahashi H, Mochizuki M, et al. Audiovestibular findings in patients with Vogt-Koyanagi-Harada disease. Acta Oto-Laryngologica. 2014;**134**(4):339-344

[37] Ozdal P, Ozdamar Y, Yazici A, Teke MY, Ozturk F. Vogt-Koyanagi-Harada disease: Clinical and demographic characteristics of patients in a specialized eye hospital in Turkey. Ocular Immunology and Inflammation. 2014;**22**(4):277-286

[38] Nakao K, Mizushima Y, Abematsu N, Goh N, Sakamoto T. Anterior ischemic optic neuropathy associated with Vogt-Koyanagi-Harada disease. Graefe's Archive for Clinical and Experimental Ophthalmology. 2009;**247**(10):1417-1425

[39] Farah ME, Costa RA, Muccioli C, Guia TA, Belfort R Jr. Photodynamic therapy with verteporfin for subfoveal choroidal neovascularization in Vogt-Koyanagi-Harada syndrome. American Journal of Ophthalmology. 2002;**134**(1):137-139

[40] Yang P, Ye Z, Xu J, Du L, Zhou Q, Qi J, et al. Macular abnormalities in Vogt-Koyanagi-Harada disease. Ocular Immunology and Inflammation. 2019;**27**(8):1195-1202

[41] Patel AK, Newcomb CW, Liesegang TL, Pujari SS, Suhler EB, Thorne JE, et al. Risk of retinal neovascularization in cases of uveitis. Ophthalmology. 2016;**123**(3):646-654

[42] Read RW, Rao NA. Utility of existing Vogt-Koyanagi-Harada syndrome diagnostic criteria at initial evaluation of the individual patient: A retrospective analysis. Ocular Immunology and Inflammation. 2000;**8**(4):227-234

[43] Read RW, Holland GN, Rao NA, Tabbara KF, Ohno S, Arellanes-Garcia L, et al. Revised diagnostic criteria for Vogt-Koyanagi-Harada disease: Report of an International Committee on Nomenclature. American Journal of Ophthalmology. 2001;**131**(5):647-652

[44] Rao NA, Gupta A, Dustin L, Chee SP, Okada AA, Khairallah M, et al. Frequency of distinguishing clinical features in Vogt-Koyanagi-Harada disease. Ophthalmology. 2010;**117**(3):591-599, 9.e1

[45] Standardization of Uveitis Nomenclature (SUN) Working Group. Classification criteria for Vogt-Koyanagi-Harada disease. American Journal of Ophthalmology. 2021;**228**:205-211

[46] Nazari H, Hariri A, Hu Z, Ouyang Y, Sadda S, Rao NA. Choroidal atrophy and loss of choriocapillaris in convalescent stage of Vogt-Koyanagi-Harada disease:

In vivo documentation. Journal of Ophthalmic Inflammation and Infection. 2014;**4**:9

[47] Parc C, Guenoun JM, Dhote R, Brézin A. Optical coherence tomography in the acute and chronic phases of Vogt-Koyanagi-Harada disease. Ocular Immunology and Inflammation. 2005;**13**(2-3):225-227

[48] Yamaguchi Y, Otani T, Kishi S. Tomographic features of serous retinal detachment with multilobular dye pooling in acute Vogt-Koyanagi-Harada disease. American Journal of Ophthalmology. 2007;**144**(2):260-265

[49] Ishihara K, Hangai M, Kita M, Yoshimura N. Acute Vogt-Koyanagi-Harada disease in enhanced spectral-domain optical coherence tomography. Ophthalmology. 2009;**116**(9):1799-1807

[50] Maruyama Y, Kishi S. Tomographic features of serous retinal detachment in Vogt-Koyanagi-Harada syndrome. Ophthalmic Surgery, Lasers & Imaging. 2004;**35**(3):239-242

[51] Shinoda K, Imamura Y, Matsumoto CS, Mizota A, Ando Y. Wavy and elevated retinal pigment epithelial line in optical coherence tomographic images of eyes with atypical Vogt-Koyanagi-Harada disease. Graefe's Archive for Clinical and Experimental Ophthalmology. 2012;**250**(9):1399-1402

[52] Nazari H, Rao NA. Resolution of subretinal fluid with systemic corticosteroid treatment in acute Vogt-Koyanagi-Harada disease. The British Journal of Ophthalmology. 2012;**96**(11):1410-1414

[53] Fong AH, Li KK, Wong D. Choroidal evaluation using enhanced depth imaging spectral-domain optical coherence tomography in Vogt-Koyanagi-Harada disease. Retina. 2011;**31**(3):502-509

[54] Yamamoto-Rodríguez L, Anduaga-Beramendi A, Mediavilla-Vallespín R, Subirà O, Garcia-Bru P, Solanich-Moreno X, et al. Automatic measurement of choroidal thickness with swept-source optical coherence tomography in chronic Vogt-Koyanagi-Harada disease: 3 years' follow-up. Journal of Ophthalmic Inflammation and Infection. 2024;**14**(1):62

[55] Maruko I, Iida T, Sugano Y, Oyamada H, Sekiryu T, Fujiwara T, et al. Subfoveal choroidal thickness after treatment of Vogt-Koyanagi-Harada disease. Retina. 2011;**31**(3):510-517

[56] Nakai K, Gomi F, Ikuno Y, Yasuno Y, Nouchi T, Ohguro N, et al. Choroidal observations in Vogt-Koyanagi-Harada disease using high-penetration optical coherence tomography. Graefe's Archive for Clinical and Experimental Ophthalmology. 2012;**250**(7):1089-1095

[57] Heussen FM, Vasconcelos-Santos DV, Pappuru RR, Walsh AC, Rao NA, Sadda SR. Ultra-wide-field green-light (532-nm) autofluorescence imaging in chronic Vogt-Koyanagi-Harada disease. Ophthalmic Surgery, Lasers & Imaging. 2011;**42**(4):272-277

[58] Koizumi H, Maruyama K, Kinoshita S. Blue light and near-infrared fundus autofluorescence in acute Vogt-Koyanagi-Harada disease. The British Journal of Ophthalmology. 2010;**94**(11):1499-1505

[59] Chee SP, Jap A, Cheung CM. The prognostic value of angiography in Vogt-Koyanagi-Harada disease. American Journal of Ophthalmology. 2010;**150**(6):888-893

[60] Huang F, Tan S, Hu J, Hu R, Yang P. Early and late treatment influence on

chorioretinal microvasculature in Vogt–Koyanagi–Harada patients using optical coherence tomography angiography. Translational Vision Science & Technology. 2024;**13**(8):15

[61] Bouchenaki N, Herbort CP. Indocyanine green angiography guided management of Vogt-Koyanagi-Harada disease. Journal of Ophthalmic and Vision Research. 2011;**6**(4):241-248

[62] Kim P, Sun HJ, Ham DI. Ultra-wide-field angiography findings in acute Vogt-Koyanagi-Harada disease. The British Journal of Ophthalmology. 2019;**103**(7):942-948

[63] Balci O, Jeannin B, Herbort CP Jr. Contribution of dual fluorescein and indocyanine green angiography to the appraisal of posterior involvement in birdshot retinochoroiditis and Vogt-Koyanagi-Harada disease. International Ophthalmology. 2018;**38**(2):527-539

[64] Yang P, Zhong Y, Du L, Chi W, Chen L, Zhang R, et al. Development and evaluation of diagnostic criteria for Vogt-Koyanagi-Harada disease. JAMA Ophthalmology. 2018;**136**(9):1025-1031

[65] Harada T, Kanbara Y, Takeuchi T, Niwa T, Majima T. Exploration of Vogt-Koyanagi-Harada syndrome by infrared choroidal angiography with indocyanine green. European Journal of Ophthalmology. 1997;**7**(2):163-170

[66] Noh H, Nam SW, Yoon JM, Ham DI. Choroidal venous overload in Vogt–Koyanagi–Harada disease. Eye (London, England). 2024;**38**(15):2960-2967

[67] Vasconcelos-Santos DV, Sohn EH, Sadda S, Rao NA. Retinal pigment epithelial changes in chronic Vogt-Koyanagi-Harada disease: Fundus autofluorescence and spectral domain-optical coherence tomography findings. Retina. 2010;**30**(1):33-41

[68] Yang P, Liu X, Zhou H, Guo W, Zhou C, Kijlstra A. Vogt-Koyanagi-Harada disease presenting as acute angle closure glaucoma at onset. Clinical & Experimental Ophthalmology. 2011;**39**(7):639-647

[69] Ling L, Gao F, Zhang Q, He T, Zhao Y, Xing Y, et al. Optical coherence tomography angiography assessed retinal and choroidal microvasculature features in patients with retinitis pigmentosa: A meta-analysis. BioMed Research International. 2019;**2019**:6723917

[70] Spaide RF, Klancnik JM Jr, Cooney MJ, Yannuzzi LA, Balaratnasingam C, Dansingani KK, et al. Volume-rendering optical coherence tomography angiography of macular telangiectasia type 2. Ophthalmology. 2015;**122**(11):2261-2269

[71] Karaca I, Yılmaz SG, Afrashi F, Nalçacı S. Assessment of macular capillary perfusion in patients with inactive Vogt-Koyanagi-Harada disease: An optical coherence tomography angiography study. Graefe's Archive for Clinical and Experimental Ophthalmology. 2020;**258**(6):1181-1190

[72] Ye X, Zhang H, Xiao P, Wang G, Hu X, Yan C, et al. Microvasculature features of Vogt-Koyanagi-Harada disease revealed by widefield swept-source optical coherence tomography angiography. Frontiers in Medicine. 2021;**8**:719593

[73] Luo K, Cai H, Hu Y, Jin C, Gan X, Deng Y, et al. Distinguishing microvasculature features of Vogt-Koyanagi-Harada in patients in acute and convalescent phases using optical coherence tomography angiography. Ocular Immunology and Inflammation. 2021;**29**(3):465-471

[74] Liang A, Jia S, Gao F, Han X, Pei M, Qu Y, et al. Decrease of choriocapillary

vascular density measured by optical coherence tomography angiography in Vogt-Koyanagi-Harada disease. Graefe's Archive for Clinical and Experimental Ophthalmology. 2021;**259**(11):3395-3404

[75] Liang A, Zhao C, Jia S, Gao F, Han X, Pei M, et al. Retinal microcirculation defects on OCTA correlate with active inflammation and vision in Vogt-Koyanagi-Harada disease. Ocular Immunology and Inflammation. 2021;**29**(7-8):1417-1423

[76] Liang R, Geng J, Jiang H, Jin S, Wang X, Liu X. Optical coherence tomography angiography in Vogt-Koyanagi-Harada patients: A systematic review and meta-analysis. Current Eye Research. 2024;**49**(9):895-904

[77] Baltmr A, Lightman S, Tomkins-Netzer O. Vogt-Koyanagi-Harada syndrome - Current perspectives. Clinical Ophthalmology. 2016;**10**:2345-2361

[78] Rothova A. Ocular involvement in sarcoidosis. The British Journal of Ophthalmology. 2000;**84**(1):110-116

[79] Lavezzo MM, Sakata VM, Morita C, Rodriguez EE, Abdallah SF, da Silva FT, et al. Vogt-Koyanagi-Harada disease: Review of a rare autoimmune disease targeting antigens of melanocytes. Orphanet Journal of Rare Diseases. 2016;**11**:29

[80] Keino H, Goto H, Mori H, Iwasaki T, Usui M. Association between severity of inflammation in CNS and development of sunset glow fundus in Vogt-Koyanagi-Harada disease. American Journal of Ophthalmology. 2006;**141**(6):1140-1142

[81] Chee SP, Jap A, Bacsal K. Spectrum of Vogt-Koyanagi-Harada disease in Singapore. International Ophthalmology. 2007;**27**(2-3):137-142

[82] Keino H, Goto H, Usui M. Sunset glow fundus in Vogt-Koyanagi-Harada disease with or without chronic ocular inflammation. Graefe's Archive for Clinical and Experimental Ophthalmology. 2002;**240**(10):878-882

[83] Jap A, Luu CD, Yeo I, Chee SP. Correlation between peripapillary atrophy and corticosteroid therapy in patients with Vogt-Koyanagi-Harada disease. Eye (London, England). 2008;**22**(2):240-245

[84] Urzua CA, Velasquez V, Sabat P, Berger O, Ramirez S, Goecke A, et al. Earlier immunomodulatory treatment is associated with better visual outcomes in a subset of patients with Vogt-Koyanagi-Harada disease. Acta Ophthalmologica. 2015;**93**(6):e475-ee80

[85] Abu El-Asrar AM, Dosari M, Hemachandran S, Gikandi PW, Al-Muammar A. Mycophenolate mofetil combined with systemic corticosteroids prevents progression to chronic recurrent inflammation and development of 'sunset glow fundus' in initial-onset acute uveitis associated with Vogt-Koyanagi-Harada disease. Acta Ophthalmologica. 2017;**95**(1):85-90

[86] Abu El-Asrar AM, Hemachandran S, Al-Mezaine HS, Kangave D, Al-Muammar AM. The outcomes of mycophenolate mofetil therapy combined with systemic corticosteroids in acute uveitis associated with Vogt-Koyanagi-Harada disease. Acta Ophthalmologica. 2012;**90**(8):e603-e608

[87] Hemady RK, Chan AS, Nguyen AT. Immunosuppressive agents and nonsteroidal anti-inflammatory drugs for ocular immune and inflammatory disorders. Ophthalmology Clinics of North America. 2005;**18**(4):511-528, vi

[88] Yang P, Ye Z, Du L, Zhou Q, Qi J, Liang L, et al. Novel treatment regimen

of Vogt-Koyanagi-Harada disease with a reduced dose of corticosteroids combined with immunosuppressive agents. Current Eye Research. 2018;**43**(2):254-261

[89] Shen E, Rathinam SR, Babu M, Kanakath A, Thundikandy R, Lee SM, et al. Outcomes of Vogt-Koyanagi-Harada disease: A subanalysis from a randomized clinical trial of antimetabolite therapies. American Journal of Ophthalmology. 2016;**168**:279-286

[90] Lescrauwaet B, Miserocchi E, Thurau S, Bodaghi B, Duchateau L, Verstraeten T, et al. Association between visual function response and reduction of inflammation in noninfectious uveitis of the posterior segment. Investigative Ophthalmology & Visual Science. 2017;**58**(9):3555-3562

[91] Acharya NR, Rathinam SR, Thundikandy R, Kanakath A, Murugan SB, Vedhanayaki R, et al. Outcomes in patients with Vogt-Koyanagi-Harada disease from the first-line antimetabolites for steroid-sparing treatment uveitis trial. American Journal of Ophthalmology. 2024;**267**:100-111

[92] Herbort CP Jr, Tugal-Tutkun I, Neri P, Pavésio C, Onal S, LeHoang P. Failure to integrate quantitative measurement methods of ocular inflammation hampers clinical practice and trials on new therapies for posterior uveitis. Journal of Ocular Pharmacology and Therapeutics. 2017;**33**(4):263-277

[93] Kim SJ, Yu HG. The use of low-dose azathioprine in patients with Vogt-Koyanagi-Harada disease. Ocular Immunology and Inflammation. 2007;**15**(5):381-387

[94] Cuchacovich M, Solanes F, Díaz G, Cermenati T, Avila S, Verdaguer J, et al. Comparison of the clinical efficacy of two different immunosuppressive regimens in patients with chronic Vogt-Koyanagi-Harada disease. Ocular Immunology and Inflammation. 2010;**18**(3):200-207

[95] Levy-Clarke G, Jabs DA, Read RW, Rosenbaum JT, Vitale A, Van Gelder RN. Expert panel recommendations for the use of anti-tumor necrosis factor biologic agents in patients with ocular inflammatory disorders. Ophthalmology. 2014;**121**(3):785-96.e3

[96] Wang Y, Gaudio PA. Infliximab therapy for 2 patients with Vogt-Koyanagi-Harada syndrome. Ocular Immunology and Inflammation. 2008;**16**(4):167-171

[97] Couto C, Schlaen A, Frick M, Khoury M, Lopez M, Hurtado E, et al. Adalimumab treatment in patients with Vogt-Koyanagi-Harada disease. Ocular Immunology and Inflammation. 2018;**26**(3):485-489

[98] Nguyen QD, Merrill PT, Jaffe GJ, Dick AD, Kurup SK, Sheppard J, et al. Adalimumab for prevention of uveitic flare in patients with inactive non-infectious uveitis controlled by corticosteroids (VISUAL II): A multicentre, double-masked, randomised, placebo-controlled phase 3 trial. Lancet. 2016;**388**(10050):1183-1192

[99] Nakai S, Takeuchi M, Usui Y, Namba K, Suzuki K, Harada Y, et al. Efficacy and safety of adalimumab for exacerbation or relapse of ocular inflammation in patients with Vogt-Koyanagi-Harada disease: A multicenter study. Ocular Immunology and Inflammation. 2024;**32**(4):367-375

[100] Rifkin LM, Birnbaum AD, Goldstein DA. TNF inhibition for ophthalmic indications: Current status and outlook. BioDrugs. 2013;**27**(4):347-357

[101] Bolletta E, Gozzi F, Mastrofilippo V, Pipitone N, De Simone L, Croci S, et al. Efficacy of rituximab treatment in Vogt-Koyanagi-Harada disease poorly controlled by traditional immunosuppressive treatment. Ocular Immunology and Inflammation. 2022;**30**(6):1303-1308

[102] Jeroudi A, Angeles-Han ST, Yeh S. Efficacy of adalimumab for pediatric Vogt-Koyanagi-Harada syndrome. Ophthalmic Surgery, Lasers & Imaging Retina. 2014;**45**(4):332-334

[103] Miserocchi E, Pontikaki I, Modorati G, Gattinara M, Meroni PL, Gerloni V. Anti-CD 20 monoclonal antibody (rituximab) treatment for inflammatory ocular diseases. Autoimmunity Reviews. 2011;**11**(1):35-39

[104] Chew SK, Levy J, Rogers S, Lim LL. Long-term outcomes of limited Vogt-Koyanagi-Harada syndrome. American Journal of Ophthalmology. 2016;**167**:52-56

[105] Ding X, Shu Q, Bai X, Chang Q, Xu G, Chen L. The role of widefield optical coherence tomography angiography in the diagnosis and management of acute Vogt-Koyanagi-Harada disease. Ocular Immunology and Inflammation. 2024;**32**(4):391-401

[106] Dick AD, Tugal-Tutkun I, Foster S, Zierhut M, Melissa Liew SH, Bezlyak V, et al. Secukinumab in the treatment of noninfectious uveitis: Results of three randomized, controlled clinical trials. Ophthalmology. 2013;**120**(4):777-787

[107] Wen J, Hu H, Chen M, Yang H, Zhao Y, Liu Y. Role of Janus kinase (JAK) inhibitor in autoimmune ocular inflammation: A systematic review. Journal of Immunology Research. 2021;**2021**:2324400

Chapter 5

Ocular Involvement in Behçet's Disease

Seher Köksaldı

Abstract

Behçet's disease is a systemic vasculitis characterized by a relapsing-remitting course and the involvement of multiple organs and systems. Ocular involvement is a hallmark of Behçet's disease and a major contributor to disease morbidity. In ophthalmology, it is a significant cause of vision-threatening inflammation, manifesting as uveitis. The primary objective of treatment is to achieve and sustain long-term remission of the disease. The management of uveitis in Behçet's disease typically necessitates systemic immunosuppression to control disease activity and prevent irreversible damage. Emerging evidence highlights the efficacy of biologic therapies in improving disease control and enhancing the quality of life for patients with uveitis. Fluorescein angiography remains the primary method for detecting active inflammation and vascular leakage, playing a key role in disease staging and prognosis. Multimodal imaging is a cornerstone in managing ocular Behçet's disease, offering invaluable tools for accurate diagnosis, personalized treatment strategies, and long-term monitoring of disease progression and therapy effectiveness.

Keywords: Behcet's disease, biologic agents, optical coherence tomography, optical coherence tomography angiography, uveitis

1. Introduction

Behçet's disease (BD) is an autoinflammatory disorder that predominantly affects the mucocutaneous, ocular, urogenital, vascular, and gastrointestinal systems. Genetic factors (human leukocyte antigen [HLA]-B51), infectious agents, heat shock proteins, abnormalities in the innate immune system—such as neutrophil hyperfunction and an increase in $\gamma\delta$ T cells—along with pro-coagulatory factors, play a crucial role [1].

Ocular manifestations, particularly fundus vascular lesions, are among the most common symptoms, occurring in nearly 70% of patients with BD [2]. A hallmark of Behçet's uveitis is vasculitis, which can affect arteries, veins, and capillaries. Its clinical manifestations include periphlebitis, macular ischemia, vascular occlusion, retinal or optic disc neovascularization, and areas of retinal non-perfusion [3, 4].

Behçet's disease lacks a definitive diagnostic test, and its diagnosis relies on identifying clinical features that conform to internationally established diagnostic criteria. According to the criteria established by the International Study Group in 1990, the diagnosis of BD requires the presence of oral ulcers along with at least two of the following four key features: recurrent genital ulcers, ocular lesions, characteristic skin lesions, and a positive pathergy test (**Table 1**) [5]. In 2014, the International Team for the Revision of the International Criteria for Behçet's Disease updated the diagnostic criteria based on new research. The revised criteria include oral aphthosis, genital aphthosis, ocular lesions (anterior uveitis, posterior uveitis, or retinal vasculitis), neurological manifestations, skin lesions (pseudofolliculitis, skin aphthosis, or erythema nodosum), and vascular manifestations (arterial thrombosis, large vein thrombosis, phlebitis, or superficial phlebitis). Each manifestation was assigned a specific point value, with oral aphthosis, genital aphthosis, and ocular lesions receiving two points each, while skin lesions, vascular manifestations, and neurological manifestations were assigned one point each. A total score of 4 or more was required for a diagnosis of BD, providing a more structured and quantitative approach to its classification (**Table 2**) [6].

The disease is observed worldwide, with the highest prevalence and often greater severity reported in countries along the historical Silk Road [7]. Behçet's disease typically manifests between the ages of 20 and 40, with onset before the age of 25 often linked to a higher risk of ocular involvement [8]. The condition is known to be particularly aggressive in young males from the far East [9]. While BD has traditionally been regarded as sporadic, instances of familial clustering have been reported, indicating a possible genetic susceptibility to the condition [10].

The HLA-B51 allele holds significant importance in regions where BD is prevalent, influencing its incidence and severity. Carriers of the HLA-B51 allele exhibit a markedly higher incidence rate of BD, with a 55% prevalence among carriers compared to 10–15% in non-carriers. Furthermore, the allele is associated with more severe clinical

Oral ulcers PLUS any two of the following features:
• Genital ulcers
• Uveitis (typical defined eye lesions)
• Typical defined skin lesions
• Positive pathergy test

Table 1.
International study group criteria for the diagnosis of Behçet's disease.

Sign/symptom	Points
Ocular lesions	2
Genital aphthosis	2
Oral aphthosis	2
Skin lesions	1
Neurological manifestations	1
Vascular manifestations	1
Positive pathergy test	1

Table 2.
International criteria for Behçet's disease (scoring ≥4 indicates Behçet's diagnosis).

manifestations, particularly posterior uveitis and neuro-Behçet, highlighting its role in disease progression and complications. Similar to its role in systemic manifestations, the HLA-B51 allele is significantly associated with a more severe form of ocular BD, occurring in 51% of affected individuals with the allele, compared to 31% in those without it [11].

2. Clinical features

The eye is the most frequently involved organ in BD with uveitis—a potentially sight-threatening condition—being one of its primary manifestations [12]. Uveitis is reported to occur in 60–80% of individuals diagnosed with BD [13]. Although there are no pathognomonic features, uveitis in BD typically manifests as acute onset hypopyon and occlusive retinal vasculitis, with inflammation predominantly affecting the retinal veins rather than the arterioles. While uveitis associated with BD is generally bilateral, inflammatory flares often occur unilaterally and alternate between the eyes [7, 14]. The disease is characterized by recurrent episodes of inflammation and spontaneous resolution of acute inflammatory symptoms within days to weeks. This unique pattern is one of the most valuable features for distinguishing Behçet's uveitis (BU) from other uveitic conditions [15].

The common anterior ocular findings include recurrent iridocyclitis, hypopyon, posterior synechiae, and peripheral anterior synechiae. Notably, hypopyon is a hallmark feature of ocular inflammatory episodes and is observed in 30–40% of cases [16]. Non-granulomatous acute iridocyclitis without hypopyon represents the most common manifestation of anterior segment inflammation in BD and is typically observed in conjunction with posterior segment inflammation. A fibrinous reaction is rare in Behçet's iridocyclitis, with freely circulating cells being the more characteristic presentation. In these cases, a smooth-layered hypopyon rapidly forms when the patient is upright. This hypopyon dissolves or shifts freely with changes in head position [15].

Only about 10% of patients, predominantly women, experience isolated episodes of anterior uveitis. The intensity and frequency of uveitis episodes can vary throughout the disease and may differ between the two eyes. The anterior and/or posterior segments of the eye can be affected either unilaterally or bilaterally, with a wide range of ocular lesions potentially occurring during the disease progression [15].

Although both the anterior and posterior segments of the eye are ultimately affected in most patients with BU, common sight-threatening ocular complications include retinal and/or optic disc edema, non-perfusion, neovascularization, and atrophy [17]. Retinal vasculitis, reported in up to 89% of cases, is the characteristic feature of BU and is recognized as a cause of retinal neovascularization, which may occur with or without retinal vessel occlusion [18]. It can affect vessels of all sizes, primarily involving veins. Retinal vasculitis is typically observed on fundoscopy as fluffy, gliotic, dry white sheaths encasing the venules (periphlebitis). The presence of multiple deep intraretinal hemorrhages, often associated with a frosted branch appearance, is a hallmark of the occlusive retinal vasculitis observed in BD [12, 19]. Central retinal artery occlusion is exceedingly rare. The disappearance of boundaries in the optic disc indicates the involvement of the optic nerve. This condition may present as isolated papillitis or as a clinical manifestation of sagittal sinus thrombosis, reflecting neurological involvement [20]. Papillitis is reported to be seen in approximately 5% of patients with BU [18].

Although infrequent, retinal neovascularization is a critical ocular manifestation, often resulting in vision-threatening complications such as vitreous hemorrhage, vitreous contraction, neovascular glaucoma, and traction retinal detachment [21]. White retinal ghost vessels, associated with optic atrophy, are observed in the end stage of the disease, indicating significant prior recurrent attacks [22].

Vitritis of varying intensity is commonly observed in over 85% of BD cases. The vitritis is typically diffuse, characterized by cellular and protein infiltration throughout the vitreous body. Vitreous precipitates may develop on the surface of the inferior peripheral retina a few days after the onset of the inflammatory attack. These vitreous precipitates, distinct from the snowballs seen in intermediate uveitis, are highly suggestive of BD [12].

Common ocular complications include secondary cataracts (38.5%), glaucoma (13%), vitreous hemorrhage (2-3%), chorioretinal and optic disc atrophy (23%),

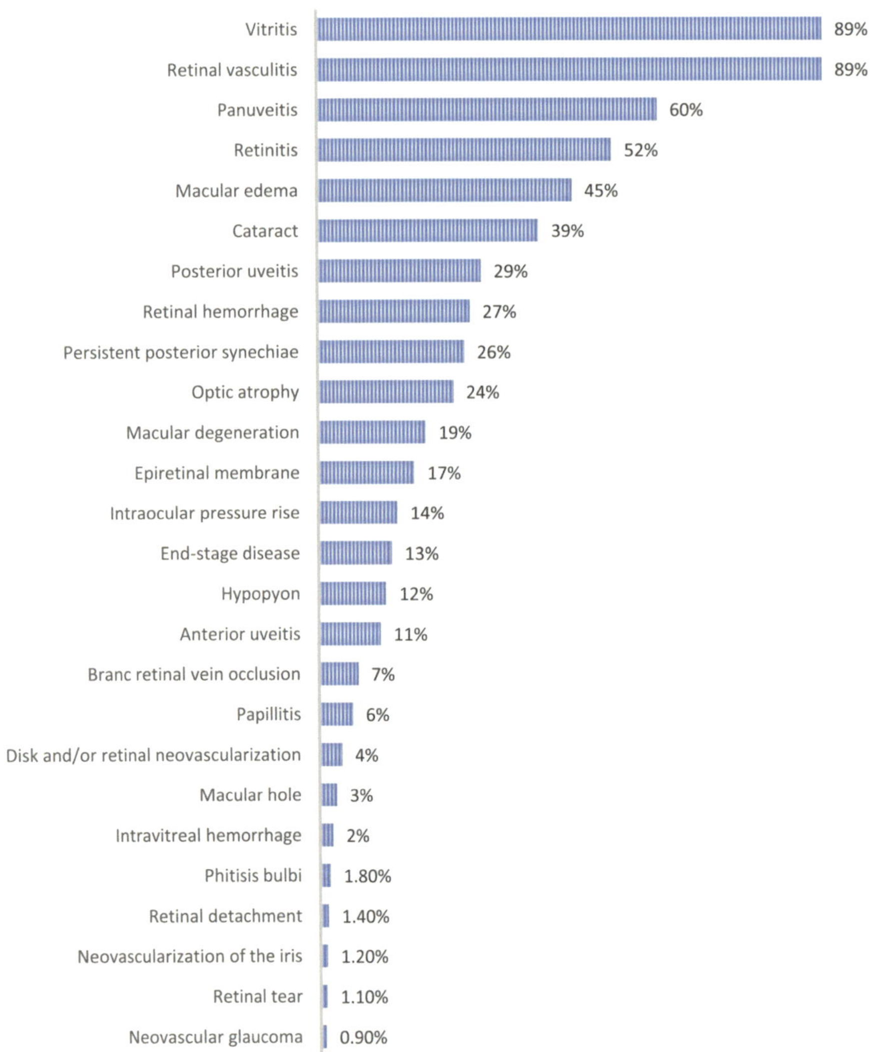

Figure 1.
The prevalence of ocular manifestations in Behçet's uveitis.

retinal detachment (1.4%), macular edema (44.5%), and ocular hypotony or phthisis bulbi (1.8%) [18]. Notably, macular edema may occur even without active ocular inflammation [23]. Epiretinal membranes are frequently associated with posterior segment inflammation, resulting in fibrosis, particularly in the macular region. Macular holes primarily arise from inflammation concentrated in the macula and fibrous adhesions between the posterior vitreous and retina, leading to the formation of either complete or incomplete macular holes [20].

Other, less common ocular manifestations of BD include episcleritis, scleritis, conjunctival ulcers, keratitis, orbital inflammatory disease, isolated optic neuritis, and oculomotor palsies [12].

The prevalence of ocular manifestations in patients with BU is summarized in **Figure 1**.

3. Imaging techniques

3.1 Color fundus photography

Fundus photography serves as a fundamental tool for visualizing intraocular lesions. It facilitates accurate documentation of lesions, enables comparative analysis during follow-up visits, and aids in monitoring lesion progression and response to treatment over time [11, 24]. Fundus photography is useful to document the retinitis foci, epiretinal membrane, macular edema, and retinal and/or neovascularization, along with the grade of vitreous haze, which is an indicator of inflammatory activity in BU (**Figures 2** and **3**) [25].

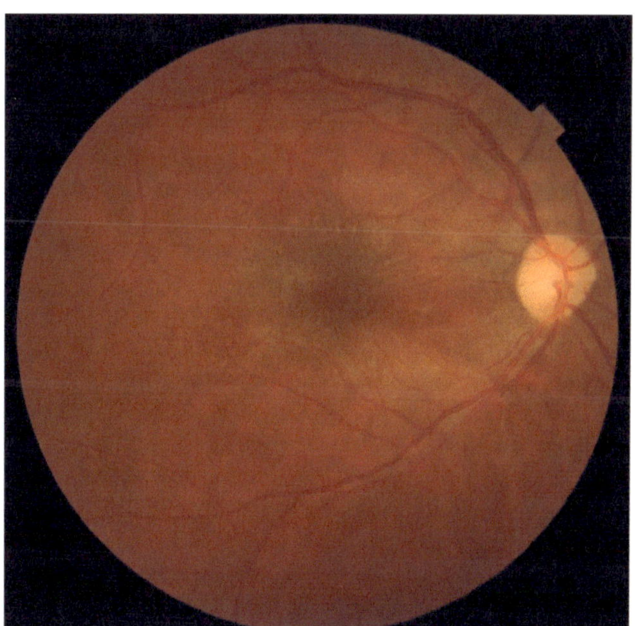

Figure 2.
Color fundus image of the right eye of a 46-year-old male patient with Behçet's disease demonstrating epiretinal membrane and cystoid macular edema (Courtesy of Ceren Durmaz Engin, MD).

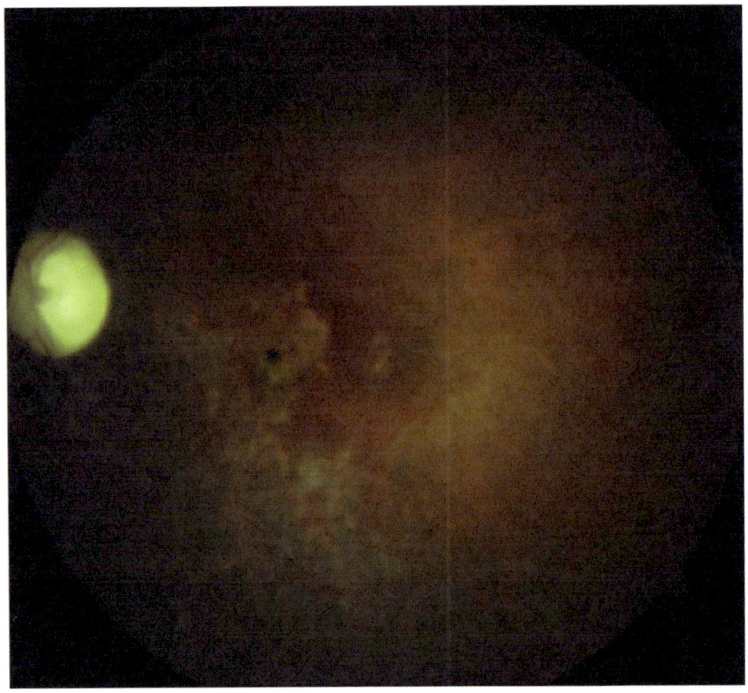

Figure 3.
Color fundus image of the left eye of a 37-year-old male patient demonstrating the end-stage disease with pale optic disc, retinal atrophy, pigmentary changes, and ghost vessels (Courtesy of Ali Osman Saatci, MD).

3.2 Fluorescein angiography

Fluorescein angiography (FA), introduced in 1962, remains the gold standard for detecting acute inflammatory lesions and occlusive disease in inflammatory retinal disorders. Fluorescein angiography commonly reveals hyperfluorescence of the optic disc, vascular dye leakage from retinal capillaries, and staining of retinal vessels due to retinal perivasculitis. These findings may be present even in eyes without ophthalmoscopic signs of clinically detectable retinal perivasculitis. Furthermore, retinal non-perfusion areas caused by retinal vasculitic occlusion and dye leakage from neovascularization at the optic disc or ischemic retinal lesions are the characteristic angiographic features observed in patients with ocular BD [23].

Eyes with a subclinically elevated anterior chamber flare, as measured by laser flare photometry, have a higher risk of recurrent uveitis attacks. This finding is associated with persistent vascular leakage observed on FA [26]. Fluorescein angiography is an indispensable tool for identifying and monitoring large retinal vessel occlusions, capillary non-perfusion, shunt vessels, and neovascularization. In eyes with disc neovascularization, distinguishing between diffuse capillary leakage and extensive capillary non-perfusion is critical for determining the appropriate treatment approach. Furthermore, FA findings such as disc neovascularization, macular window defects, and macular ischemia are strongly associated with poor visual outcomes in patients with active BU [27, 28].

Diffuse vascular leakage in a fern-like pattern is the characteristic finding in BD and is commonly observed during the chronic phases of inflammation. This pattern is typically identified through FA, where it appears as a diffuse, fern-like leakage

DOI: http://dx.doi.org/10.5772/intechopen.1009801

from the retinal capillaries [29]. Retinal vasculitis is characterized angiographically by an apparent enlargement of the vascular caliber, staining of the retinal vessels, and late-phase leakage. These changes may present as focal, multifocal, or diffuse patterns, involving both large and small vessels, particularly the veins and capillaries of the optic disc, as well as the posterior and/or peripheral retina [12]. Persistent capillary leakage following the resolution of clinical inflammatory signs indicates an inadequate therapeutic response (**Figures 4** and 5) [19].

3.3 Indocyanine green angiography

Indocyanine green angiography (ICGA) can be employed in the selected cases, particularly when it is necessary to exclude primary choroidal inflammatory conditions. It is also valuable in confirming the diagnosis of central serous chorioretinopathy, which may occur due to high-dose corticosteroid therapy in patients with Behçet's disease [25]. Indocyanine green angiography is utilized to assess choroidal involvement in posterior segment inflammation, and it reveals leakage from choroidal vessels as well as hypofluorescent and hyperfluorescent lesions [20]. However, the utility of ICGA in current clinical practice remains limited [30].

3.4 Optical coherence tomography

Optical coherence tomography (OCT) offers critical insights into macular anatomy, including the location and extent of vitreomacular traction, the presence of subretinal or intraretinal fluid, the formation of a macular hole or atrophy, and the structural integrity of photoreceptors, as well as the middle and inner retinal nuclear and plexiform layers. These findings can assist in differentiating between reversible and irreversible causes of vision loss [17]. Optical coherence tomography is most commonly utilized for the detection and management of cystoid macular edema,

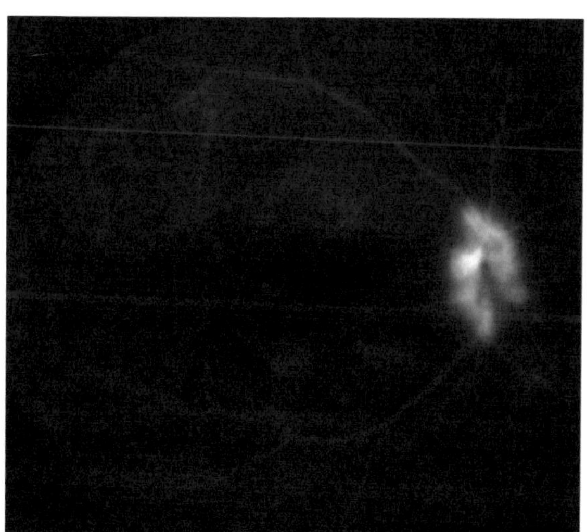

Figure 4.
Late-phase fluorescein angiography of the right eye of a 29-year-old male patient demonstrating dye leakage from capillaries in the macular and mid-peripheral region, as well as from optic disc, indicating neovascularization. (Courtesy of Ali Osman Saatci, MD).

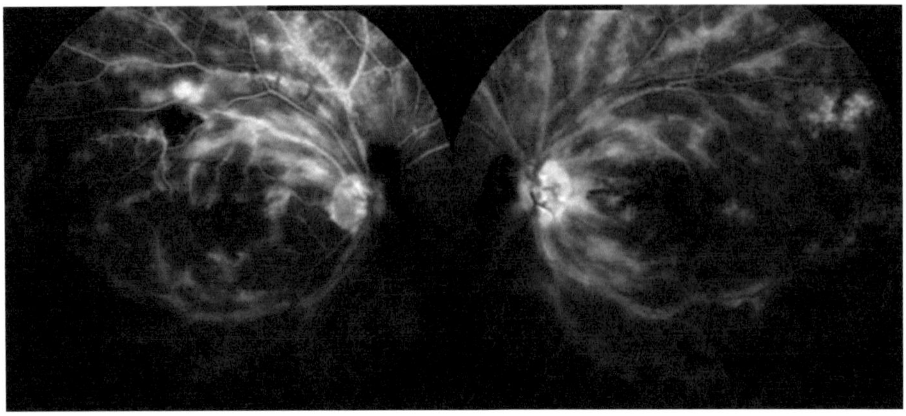

Figure 5.
Fluorescein angiography images of both eyes of a 30-year-old male patient demonstrate diffuse, fern-like dye leakage, non-perfusion, and hypofluorescent areas due to retinal hemorrhage and retinitis foci (Courtesy of Ali Osman Saatci, MD).

for documenting non-glaucomatous retinal nerve fiber layer defects linked to inner retinal atrophy following focal infarcts, and for screening glaucomatous or non-glaucomatous optic atrophy by automated comparison with the reference standards (**Figure 6**) [31].

3.5 Optical coherence tomography angiography

Optical coherence tomography angiography is a non-invasive imaging modality that provides a three-dimensional mapping of the retinal and choroidal microcirculation. In BU, various macular microvascular alterations have been identified, predominantly affecting the deep retinal capillary plexus. These include capillary hypoperfusion, dilation and shunting, disruption of the capillary network architecture, enlargement of the foveal avascular zone, and a reduction in capillary density [32].

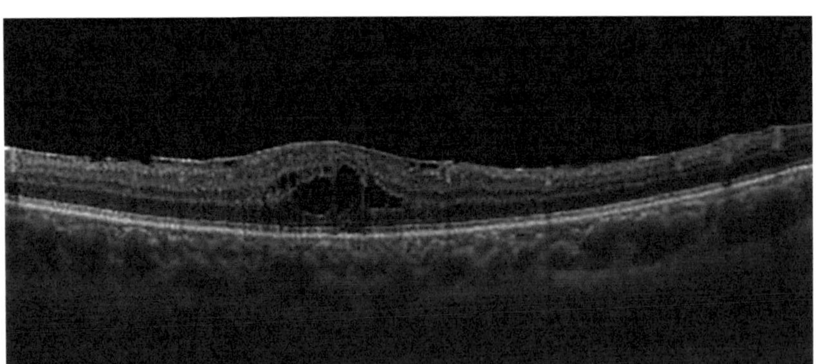

Figure 6.
Transfoveal swept-source optical coherence tomographic section of the right eye of a 46-year-old male patient with Behçet's disease demonstrating epiretinal membrane, intraretinal cysts, disruption of the retinal layers, and occasional posterior vitreous cells. (Courtesy of Ceren Durmaz Engin, MD).

4. Differential diagnosis

The differential diagnosis of occlusive retinal vasculitis in BU encompasses several conditions that can present with similar clinical findings, including retinal vein occlusion, retinal artery occlusion, sarcoidosis, Susac's syndrome, and systemic lupus erythematosus. Differentiating BU from these disorders is crucial for appropriate management, as each condition has distinct underlying pathophysiological mechanisms and treatment approaches. A detailed comparison of the distinctive ocular, FA, and systemic features of these disorders is summarized in **Table 3**.

5. Treatment options

The main goals in managing patients with BU are to quickly resolve intraocular inflammation, prevent recurrent flare-ups, and achieve complete remission while preserving vision. Previously, the only treatment options for BD were systemic corticosteroids and various immunosuppressive drugs. However, these treatments often fail to provide long-term remission, especially in cases of ocular involvement. The development of new biologic drugs has now transformed the treatment approach for BD [33].

Condition	Ocular features	Fluorescein angiographic findings	Systemic associations
Behçet's disease	Bilateral retinal vasculitis affecting both arteries and veins, often with hypopyon uveitis	Diffuse fern-like capillary leakage, optic disc hyperfluorescence, and areas of non-perfusion	Mucocutaneous ulcers, arthritis, central nervous system involvement
Retinal vein occlusion	Unilateral dilated and tortuous veins, retinal hemorrhages, and macular edema	Delayed venous filling, peripheral ischemia, and collateral vessel formation in chronic cases	Hypertension, diabetes, and hypercoagulable states
Retinal artery occlusion	Sudden vision loss, a cherry-red spot at the fovea, and attenuated arteries	Delayed arterial filling without leakage and box-carring blood flow pattern	Carotid artery disease, cardiac emboli, and systemic vasculitis
Sarcoidosis	Periphlebitis, multifocal chorioretinitis, and candle-wax drippings along veins	Segmental venous leakage and choroidal granulomas	Pulmonary involvement and elevated angiotensin-converting enzyme levels
Susac's syndrome	Branch retinal artery occlusion, Gass plaques	Multifocal arterial occlusions without significant leakage	Hearing loss, encephalopathy, white matter lesions on magnetic resonance imaging
Systemic lupus erythematosus	Retinal hemorrhages, cotton wool spots	Diffuse vascular leakage and capillary dropout	Nephritis, joint inflammation

Table 3.
Differential diagnosis of occlusive retinal vasculitis in uveitis.

5.1 Corticosteroids

Systemic corticosteroids are highly effective for rapidly controlling acute ocular inflammation while waiting for immunosuppressive medication to take full effect. Oral corticosteroid therapy should begin with prednisone or prednisolone at a dose of 1 mg/kg/day. In severe cases, such as retinal vasculitis or optic neuropathy, initial treatment may involve intravenous methylprednisolone at 1 g daily for 3 days before transitioning to oral corticosteroids [34].

Managing BU typically requires high doses of corticosteroids to maintain remission, and it is widely recognized that long-term use of these drugs can lead to significant and undesirable side effects [35]. High-dose corticosteroid treatment for an acute episode should last no longer than 2 to 4 weeks. Following this, the dosage should be reduced gradually by approximately 10% every 1 to 2 weeks. The goal is either complete discontinuation, if achievable, or a maintenance dose of ≤5–7.5 mg/day. As the steroid dose decreases, tapering should proceed more slowly with longer intervals to ensure safety [34].

5.2 Antimetabolites

5.2.1 Methotrexate

Methotrexate is a folate analog that inhibits dihydrofolate reductase, thereby blocking the synthesis of tetrahydrofolate and disrupting nucleic acid and protein synthesis. The dosage regimen for methotrexate in BU treatment follows the same oral protocol as for rheumatoid arthritis. Treatment typically begins with a dose of 15 mg/week, gradually increasing to a target dose of 25 mg/week, depending on patient tolerance. Once the disease stabilizes, the maintenance dose is reduced to 15 mg/week [36].

Common adverse effects of methotrexate include bone marrow suppression, hepatotoxicity, pulmonary toxicity, gastrointestinal disturbances, alopecia, and dermatitis. To minimize the risk of hematological disorders and other complications, it is essential to supplement with folic acid (1 mg/day) or folinic acid and to regularly monitor blood counts and liver function during treatment. Methotrexate can also reduce sperm count in men, typically requiring more than 3 months to return to normal after discontinuation. Due to its teratogenic effects, methotrexate is contraindicated in pregnant and lactating women [36].

Research on intravitreal methotrexate for BU treatment is limited, and its effectiveness and safety require further investigation. Close monitoring is necessary for potential adverse effects, including corneal endothelial damage and decompensation [37, 38].

5.2.2 Azathioprine

Azathioprine is an antimetabolite with cytostatic properties that target dividing cells [12]. Azathioprine at a dose of 2.5 mg/kg/day, in combination with corticosteroids (level of recommendation 1b), is recommended as the first-line treatment for ocular BD affecting the posterior segment. However, in refractory cases characterized by a significant decline in visual acuity (greater than two lines on a 10/10 scale) and/or retinal involvement (such as macular involvement or retinal vasculitis), treatment should include either cyclosporine-A or infliximab alongside azathioprine and corticosteroids [39].

It typically requires 2 to 3 months to achieve its full therapeutic effect. Therefore, concurrent use of corticosteroids is recommended to provide rapid and effective control of acute inflammatory episodes during the initial phase of azathioprine treatment. Once inflammation is well-controlled with a low maintenance dose of corticosteroids, the azathioprine dosage is gradually reduced by 12.5 mg every 3 months. Discontinuation may be achieved after 18 months to 2 years; however, in many cases, a longer duration of treatment is required [6]. Due to its potential hematologic and hepatic toxicity, regular monitoring of complete blood counts and liver enzyme levels is essential during the treatment [12].

5.2.3 Mycophenolate mofetil/mycophenolate sodium

Mycophenolate mofetil has demonstrated efficacy as a corticosteroid-sparing agent in uncontrolled studies on noninfectious uveitis, including cases of BD-associated uveitis. Additionally, a report documented its long-term beneficial effects in four patients with parenchymal neuro-Behçet disease who were either intolerant or unresponsive to other therapeutic agents [40]. Furthermore, mycophenolate sodium is preferred due to its improved tolerability, primarily attributed to a lower incidence of gastrointestinal side effects [41].

For BU treatment, mycophenolate mofetil is usually given orally at a dose of 0.5–2 g/day or 10–30 mg/kg/day. The typical starting dose is 500 mg twice daily, which is gradually increased to the target dose of 1000–1500 mg twice daily, depending on the patient's tolerance [42]. Mycophenolate mofetil is frequently combined with low-dose corticosteroids or calcineurin inhibitors, such as cyclosporine and tacrolimus, and has demonstrated good therapeutic efficacy. Since mycophenolate mofetil has a mechanism of action similar to azathioprine, co-administration of the two is not recommended [43]. Mycophenolate mofetil can cause gastrointestinal side effects, such as nausea, vomiting, diarrhea, and loss of appetite, which can be alleviated by administering mycophenolate mofetil suspension. Additionally, mycophenolate mofetil may lead to less common adverse effects, including liver and kidney toxicity, bone marrow suppression, and an increased risk of infections and tumors, requiring careful monitoring [44].

5.3 Alkylating agents

Alkylating agents alter lymphocyte DNA by inducing cross-linking, which disrupts DNA replication and transcription, resulting in cell death and a reduction in T/B cell counts. This subsequently impairs both humoral and cellular immunities [36]. The limited use of alkylating agents in BD-associated uveitis is attributed to the lack of controlled trials and their potential for severe adverse effects, including an increased risk of malignancy [41]. Cyclophosphamide and chlorambucil are the main alkylating agents used in BU treatment. However, due to their comparable pharmacological actions, combining them is not recommended [36].

5.3.1 Cyclophosphamide

Cyclophosphamide is a highly effective anti-inflammatory medication, particularly beneficial in cases of retinal vasculitis where immediate inflammatory control is required. Its use in the management of mucocutaneous BD was first introduced in the late 1960s, with its application in ocular BD being reported in 1984. The recommended initial oral dose of cyclophosphamide for BU treatment is typically between 1 and 2 mg/kg/day, followed by a maintenance dose of 1 mg/kg/day [36]. For patients who experience severe retinal vasculitis or hemorrhagic cystitis following oral cyclophosphamide treatment, high-dose intravenous pulse therapy may be considered. In this case, the drug is typically administered intravenously at a dose of 1 g per month, often in combination with other immunomodulatory therapies [45].

Cyclophosphamide is metabolized by the liver and kidneys, with acrolein, a metabolite, potentially causing hemorrhagic cystitis and bladder tumors. Adequate hydration can help prevent and alleviate these effects. Common adverse effects of cyclophosphamide, including leukopenia, liver damage, and fertility impairment, are dose-dependent and typically occur at doses used in BU treatment [46]. Cyclophosphamide should be discontinued if the white blood cell count falls below 2.5/L. The most adverse effects are reversible, and intravenous administration can help decrease both the frequency and severity of these effects [44].

5.3.2 Chlorambucil

Chlorambucil's mechanism of action is similar to cyclophosphamide, though it tends to have a milder, longer-lasting effect and fewer severe side effects. As a result, chlorambucil is an effective treatment option for BU patients who do not respond to cyclophosphamide. In addition to managing uveitis and extraocular symptoms, such as oral ulcers and skin lesions in BD patients, chlorambucil is especially beneficial for those with severe extraocular manifestations, including central nervous system involvement and thrombotic venous inflammation [47].

The dosing regimen for chlorambucil in BU treatment is not yet standardized. It is important to note that chlorambucil takes longer to show its effects, often requiring more than 2 months to reach its full impact. Therefore, the lack of noticeable efficacy in the early stages of treatment does not necessarily suggest that the drug is ineffective. Treatment should be continued for a minimum of 3 to 5 months to assess its effectiveness. The adverse effects of chlorambucil are similar cyclophosphamide and include bone marrow suppression, gonadal dysfunction, liver and kidney damage, and gastrointestinal symptoms. Prolonged use of chlorambucil may result in a reduction in sperm count or even azoospermia in men, usually after 4 months of treatment, and may induce menopause or amenorrhea in women over the age of 35 [36].

5.4 Calcineurin inhibitors/T-cell inhibitors

5.4.1 Cyclosporine A

Cyclosporine is a T-lymphocyte inhibitor that inhibits calcineurin. Since its introduction in the 1980s, it has represented a significant improvement in visual prognosis [48]. The initial recommended dose is 2 to 5 mg/kg/day, divided into two doses. This dose should be maintained until long-term control of inflammation is achieved with a low-dose corticosteroid regimen. A gradual tapering of cyclosporine is essential, reducing the dose by 10% every 2 to 3 months, to minimize the risk of rebound inflammation upon discontinuation [12]. The combination of cyclosporine with low-dose prednisone yields a favorable response with reduced toxicity. This treatment has also been shown to be beneficial for skin, mucosal, ear, throat, and nose lesions, as well as for thrombophlebitis. Cyclosporine-A is associated with side effects, notably nephrotoxicity and hypertension. As such, regular monitoring of serum creatinine levels and blood pressure is required. Additionally, cyclosporine-A is contraindicated in neuro-Behçet's disease due to its potential neurotoxic effects [49]. Other frequent adverse effects include gingival hyperplasia, hypertrichosis, acroparesthesias, and cholestatic hepatitis. Prolonged use has been linked to an elevated risk of cholestatic hepatitis, lymphoproliferative syndromes, and malignant skin tumors [12].

5.4.2 Tacrolimus

The efficacy of tacrolimus is promising, with 67% of patients achieving stable disease control following a switch from cyclosporine-A, and 75% of treatment-naive cases achieving stable disease control [50]. Administered in two divided doses at a range of 0.05 to 0.20 mg/kg/day, this product offers similar efficacy to cyclosporine-A. However, it carries a higher risk of side effects, such as hypertension, nephrotoxicity, gastrointestinal toxicity, and diabetes [51].

5.5 Other

5.5.1 Colchicine

Colchicine, administered at a dosage of 1–2 mg/day, is another anti-inflammatory medication commonly utilized in the management of BD, with its use dating back to the 1980s. This medication has been reported to serve as a valuable adjunctive therapy, capable of reducing disease severity while being associated with the fewer adverse effects compared to corticosteroid therapy. However, although colchicine demonstrates significant efficacy in the treating oral and cutaneous ulcers, it is not effective in managing ocular or articular inflammation [19, 52].

5.6 Biological agents

5.6.1 Tumor necrosis factor inhibitors

Tumor necrosis factor (TNF) is a multifunctional cytokine primarily produced by monocytes, macrophages, and T-lymphocytes. In response to infection or immunological injury, it is also synthesized to a lesser extent by neutrophils and mast cells. Tumor necrosis factor promotes inflammation through both direct cytotoxic effects and various indirect mechanisms. These include the regulation of other pro-inflammatory cytokines, the release of arachidonic acid-derived mediators, reactive oxygen and nitrogen species, metalloproteinases, chemokines, adhesion molecules, and factors involved in angiogenesis [13]. The neutralization of TNF activity in clinical practice leads to the suppression of the pro-inflammatory cytokine cascade. Consequently, there is reduced recruitment of inflammatory cells from the bloodstream to the site of inflammation, decreased angiogenesis driven by vascular endothelial growth factor, and modulation of chemokines, acute phase proteins, and vascular permeability [53].

In 2004, the first case series was published, reporting the efficacy of TNF-α blockers in treating uveitis [54]. In recent years, clinical studies have demonstrated elevated concentrations of TNF and soluble TNF receptors in the serum and/or aqueous humor of patients with BD, particularly during phases of increased disease activity [55].

Anti-TNF-α therapy effectively suppresses nearly all manifestations of the disease, yielding an immediate and significant clinical response [13].

5.6.1.1 Infliximab

Infliximab is a chimeric monoclonal IgG1κ antibody, composed of murine and human regions, that binds to both circulating and membrane-bound TNF-α. It is administered *via* intravenous infusion [13]. Infliximab was officially approved in Japan in 2007 for treating BD complicated by refractory uveoretinitis that does not respond to conventional therapies [21].

It is administered intravenously at a dosage of 3–5 mg/kg at weeks 0, 2, and 6, followed by an administration every 8 weeks. The half-life of infliximab is approximately 10 days, although its downstream biological effects can persist for up to 8 weeks [56]. Infliximab demonstrates a shorter time to respond in this context compared to other immunosuppressive regimens, including interferon, which has been reported to produce a response within a range of 11 days to 24 weeks [57].

Long-term use of infliximab therapy for BU may lead to the development of acquired resistance. Despite receiving infliximab treatment, a subset of patients experiences recurrent uveitis. When starting infliximab treatment, it is important to gradually taper off or administer previous immunosuppressive agents at lower doses. This approach may help prevent the recurrence of uveitis during the first 5–6 months of treatment. The concomitant use of other immunosuppressive agents alongside infliximab has been recommended to reduce the risk of developing human anti-chimeric antibodies or antibodies against infliximab. Monitoring human anti-chimeric antibodies in patient serum can provide direct insight into this issue [58].

Infliximab has also proven effective in treating extraocular manifestations, including oral and genital ulcers and/or arthritis, in most patients [59]. Additional case series and reports have suggested that patients with severe mucocutaneous lesions demonstrate rapid and substantial responses to infliximab therapy, most administered at doses of 3 or 5 mg/kg [60, 61].

Serious adverse effects associated with infliximab therapy have been reported, including an increased risk of malignancies, tuberculosis, multiple sclerosis, optic neuritis, congestive heart failure, and lupus-like reactions. Furthermore, pulmonary embolism and coronary artery thrombosis have also been observed during infliximab treatment. Since BD is often linked with neurological manifestations and thrombosis, these potential risks must be carefully considered in patients with a history of these predispositions [13].

5.6.1.2 Adalimumab

Adalimumab, an anti-TNF agent administered subcutaneously, has been successfully used to treat refractory uveitis, as well as BD-associated refractory panuveitis and retinal vasculitis [21]. Adalimumab is given *via* subcutaneous injection at a dosage of 40 mg every 1 to 2 weeks. It is recommended as the primary treatment for ocular involvement in BD [62].

Adalimumab is approved by the EMA and FDA for the treating non-infectious intermediate, posterior, and panuveitis, including that associated with BD. As a fully humanized antibody, adalimumab is associated with a lower risk of developing autoantibodies and allergic reactions. The side effects are generally like those of infliximab. A key advantage of adalimumab is its subcutaneous administration, which may improve patient compliance and allow for stable serum concentrations.

The initial report on the use of ADA therapy for BU was published in 2007. Mushtaq et al. [63] reported three patients with sight-threatening BU, initially managed with infliximab, who were switched to adalimumab due to difficulties attending infusion appointments. All three patients successfully maintained disease remission and visual acuity without relapse [63]. Adalimumab has proven effective in treating uveitis related to BD, resulting in improved visual acuity, reduced reliance on steroids and immunosuppressants, and long-term remission [12, 64].

5.6.1.3 Etanercept

Experience with etanercept is limited, so it should be reserved for patients who cannot tolerate infliximab or adalimumab. Regarding side effects, treatment has been linked to a higher risk of infections and the emergence of autoimmune diseases. Additionally, there are reports of invasive opportunistic fungal infections, tuberculosis reactivation, and the potential for inducing or worsening demyelinating and lymphoproliferative disorders [62].

5.6.1.4 Golimumab

Golimumab is a monoclonal anti-TNF-α therapy that has been approved for the treatment of rheumatoid arthritis and ankylosing spondylitis. In retinal vasculitis, golimumab has proven effective in controlling active inflammation and reducing the incidence of relapses [19].

It is administered subcutaneously at a dosage of 50 mg once a month. Due to its molecular structure as a fully human monoclonal antibody, golimumab has a lower likelihood of developing neutralizing antibodies compared to other anti-TNF agents. However, despite being fully human, resistance to golimumab may still develop. Other advantages of golimumab therapy over other TNF antagonists include its reduced dosing schedule, as it is administered once a month through subcutaneous self-injection [33].

5.6.2 Specific receptor antagonists

5.6.2.1 Canakinumab

Canakinumab is a fully human monoclonal antibody designed to specifically target interleukin (IL)-1β. By binding to IL-1 beta, it prevents its interaction with IL-1 receptors (IL-1RI and IL-1RII). Canakinumab, administered intravenously or subcutaneously, effectively neutralizes the bioactivity of IL-1β, a key mediator in various inflammatory disorders [65]. Early clinical trials have confirmed that administering canakinumab every 2 weeks is safe and effective. This regimen offers a significant advantage over the current treatment with the human IL-1 receptor antagonist anakinra, which necessitates daily injections and is frequently associated with poor patient tolerance [33].

5.6.2.2 Tocilizumab

Research has shown elevated IL-6 levels in the vitreous fluid of patients with chronic uveitis, not only in idiopathic cases but also in those associated with systemic inflammatory diseases such as sarcoidosis, Vogt-Koyanagi-Harada syndrome, and BD

[66, 67]. This suggests that IL-6 inhibition may be a beneficial therapeutic approach for refractory uveitis. In this regard, Deroux et al. [68] conducted the largest study on refractory BD treated with tocilizumab. Among the four patients studied, three had severe ocular involvement (relapsing posterior uveitis, bilateral posterior uveitis, and bilateral panuveitis), all of whom exhibited a remarkable response to tocilizumab. Additionally, the treatment significantly reduced corticosteroid dependence, highlighting its corticosteroid-sparing potential [68].

Hirano et al. [69] reported the first case of refractory BD successfully treated with tocilizumab, demonstrating not only uveitis improvement but also the resolution of other systemic manifestations [69]. Additionally, a severe case of neuro-BD with concurrent severe ocular involvement, initially treated with a high-frequency infliximab regimen, showed an excellent initial response but later developed IgA nephropathy. Following the switch to tocilizumab, complete remission of all clinical manifestations was achieved after the second infusion [70].

However, tocilizumab is not always effective in treating refractory ocular BD, as demonstrated by Papo et al. [71] in a study of eight consecutive patients with non-infectious uveitis [71]. Furthermore, a notable drawback of tocilizumab is its relatively limited efficacy in controlling mucocutaneous symptoms of BD, as reported by multiple experts [72, 73].

5.6.2.3 *Anakinra*

In 1993, researchers began targeting IL-1 by introducing anakinra, a recombinant form of the naturally occurring IL-1 receptor antagonist (IL-1Ra), which blocks the activity of both IL-1α and IL-1β. The adult dose of 100 mg is administered daily through subcutaneous injection [74]. In a retrospective study of nine patients with BD resistant to conventional and anti-TNF therapies, Cantarini et al. [75] found that administering the IL-1 receptor antagonist anakinra at an initial daily dose of 100 mg rapidly improved disease symptoms in seven patients, though it failed to prevent relapses. Among the four patients treated for active uveitis, three achieved complete resolution of intraocular inflammation after starting anakinra; however, relapses occurred after an average of 24 weeks. Increasing the anakinra dosage partially or completely controlled the disease in three patients. Notably, two patients developed retinal vasculitis after approximately 8 months of anakinra therapy [75]. Emmi et al. [76] reported that increasing the daily dose of anakinra or transitioning to canakinumab could facilitate disease control in patients who initially demonstrated a poor response to anakinra. Furthermore, reducing the infusion intervals may be beneficial for patients who exhibited an incomplete initial response to canakinumab 150 mg administered every 8 weeks [76].

5.6.2.4 *Gevokizumab*

Gevokizumab is a recombinant, partially humanized monoclonal antibody that binds to interleukin-1 beta, reducing its affinity for the interleukin-1 receptor type I while maintaining its affinity for the interleukin-1 receptor type II. As a modulating antibody, it does not block the assembly of the interleukin-1 beta signaling complex; instead, it downregulates interleukin-1 beta activity in cytokine release assays. With a circulating half-life of approximately 25 days, gevokizumab enables once-monthly dosing [77].

A proof-of-concept study assessed the safety and efficacy of gevokizumab in seven patients with BD, all of whom had posterior uveitis, panuveitis, and/

or retinal vasculitis that were refractory to treatment with azathioprine and/or cyclosporine. The administration of a single 0.3 mg/kg infusion of gevokizumab resulted in a rapid and sustained reduction in intraocular inflammation, enhanced visual acuity, and a decrease in anterior chamber cells and flare, vitreous haze, and retinal infiltrates. Notably, these improvements occurred despite the discontinuation of immunosuppressive treatments and without any increase in corticosteroid dosage [78]. The findings of the phase 2 exploratory study indicate that gevokizumab is both safe and well-tolerated in patients with uveitis related to BD [79].

Tugal-Tutkun et al. [80] conducted a study with 83 patients (40 receiving gevokizumab and 43 receiving a placebo). The findings indicated that gevokizumab could reduce uveitis severity, lower the incidence of macular edema, and decrease mean central macular thickness, particularly during the first 6 months of treatment, ultimately contributing to the preservation of vision [80].

5.6.2.5 Secukinumab

Secukinumab is a fully human, high-affinity monoclonal antibody that selectively binds to IL-17A, blocking downstream signaling pathways responsible for neutrophil and macrophage activation [81]. Interleukin-21 plays a crucial role in regulating Th17 and regulatory T-cells, while IL-17 production is significantly upregulated in BD patients with active uveitis [82].

The SHIELD study examined 118 patients with active uveitis due to BD to evaluate multiple outcomes. Although the primary endpoint did not reach statistical significance, secondary endpoints—such as the reduction or discontinuation of immunosuppressive medications—showed a significant difference between the secukinumab and placebo groups. However, the authors acknowledged several limitations, including the small sample size, differences in disease severity, the complex cytokine interactions unique to each patient, and potential confounding effects of concurrent immunosuppressive treatments [83].

5.6.2.6 Ustekinumab

Interleukin-23 is a heterodimeric cytokine composed of two subunits, p40 and p19, and plays a pivotal role in Th17 differentiation, promoting the production of IL-17, IL-17F, IL-6, and TNF. Given the elevated IL-23 levels observed in BD, ustekinumab—a fully human monoclonal antibody that targets the shared p40 subunit of IL-12 and IL-23—prevents their interaction with the IL-12Rβ1 receptor, effectively blocking downstream signaling pathways [82].

Among the primary manifestations of BD, anterior uveitis was observed in conjunction with psoriasis and hidradenitis suppurativa—a rare combination effectively managed with ustekinumab. According to the literature, the treatment protocol included a subcutaneous dose of 45 mg at weeks 0 and 4, followed by maintenance dosing every 12 weeks. The patient remained symptom-free and relapse-free for at least 36 months without the need for additional immunosuppressive therapy [84].

5.6.2.7 Daclizumab

Daclizumab, a humanized monoclonal antibody that targets the α-subunit (CD25) of the IL-2 receptor, has the ability to restore immune homeostasis in dysregulated systems. It binds to the high-affinity Tac-p55 protein of the IL-2 receptor, blocking IL-2 signaling in activated T-cells. Elevated serum levels of soluble IL-2R have been observed in patients with active BD [85, 86].

The most common adverse events observed were of a dermatologic nature, including eczema, fibrosis, folliculitis, and psoriasis. Additionally, solid neoplasms may develop during a prolonged follow-up period, such as skin squamous cell carcinoma, vulvar carcinoma, renal cell carcinoma, and esophageal cancer [87].

5.6.3 Lymphocyte inhibitors

5.6.3.1 Rituximab

Rituximab, a chimeric monoclonal antibody targeting CD20, has been used off-label in patients with BD [82]. The available data on rituximab in ocular BD are still limited [33]. Sadreddini et al. [88] were the first to administer rituximab in a case of BD complicated by retinal vasculitis, resulting in complete remission of ocular inflammation and a significant corticosteroid-sparing effect [88].

Davatchi et al. [89] conducted a single-blind randomized controlled trial to evaluate the effectiveness of rituximab in combination with conventional immunosuppressive therapy for refractory BU. Twenty patients with treatment-resistant BU were randomly assigned to either a rituximab group (rituximab + methotrexate + glucocorticoids) or a conventional treatment group (cyclophosphamide + azathioprine + prednisolone). After 6 months of follow-up, the rituximab group demonstrated significant improvements in uveitis, as well as reductions in retinal, optic disc, and macular edema compared to the conventional treatment group. However, no significant differences were observed in visual acuity, disease activity index for posterior uveitis and retinal vasculitis, or total inflammatory activity index [89].

5.6.3.2 Alemtuzumab

Alemtuzumab is a humanized monoclonal IgG1 antibody that targets CD52, with the well-recognized effects on CD52+ cells. Within minutes of infusion, it induces significant depletion of T and B cells through both antibody-dependent and complement-dependent cytolysis [90]. Case reports by Lockwood et al. [91] demonstrated the therapeutic effects of alemtuzumab on ocular, cutaneous, and neurological manifestations of BD [91].

The efficacy of alemtuzumab is likely attributed to its ability to induce long-term lymphopenia. Given the significant risk of infections, careful consideration is required when using this agent, which should be reserved for cases of multi-drug failure [82].

Adverse events included infections such as pneumonia and colitis caused by *Clostridium difficile*, thyroid dysfunction, autoimmune hemolytic anemia, and esophageal carcinoma [92].

5.6.4 Interferon-alpha

Interferons are a class of cytokines comprising type I interferons, including interferon-alpha (IFN-α) and interferon-beta (IFN-β), and type II interferon, IFN-γ [13]. They are naturally produced cytokines. Type I interferons can be generated by nearly all cell types; however, antigen-presenting cells, particularly plasmacytoid dendritic cells, are the primary producers, even at the early stages of the immune response. Thus, type I IFNs, especially IFN-a, are highly effective in the management of BD as well as chronic uveitic macular edema [93]. Both recombinant human IFN-α2a and IFN-α2b have been effectively employed in treating posterior uveitis, with IFN-α2a being the most widely used in most studies. IFN-α2a is reported to be more effective than IFN-α2b [57]. According to the consensus of experts from the American Uveitis Society, anti-TNF-α therapy should be considered as the first-line treatment for BD with retinal vasculitis [62].

IFN-α is administered through subcutaneous injection. Typically, treatment begins with high-dose daily injections ranging from 3.0 to 6.0 million international units (MIU) per day, followed by a tapering regimen to lower-dose intermittent injections (3.0 MIU two to three times per week) [13]. Steroids and immunosuppressive agents may counteract the effects of IFN. As a standard practice, second-line immunosuppressants are discontinued before initiating IFN-α therapy, and many ophthalmologists also reduce corticosteroid doses to the lowest possible level [94]. Other treatment protocols have utilized initial lower doses of IFN-α (3.0–4.5 million international units three times weekly) in conjunction with high doses of prednisone, resulting in the successful management of uveitis [13, 95].

The therapeutic response to IFN-α in BU has been observed within 2 weeks for the resolution of retinal infiltrates and 4 weeks for the control of vasculitis, macular edema, and activity in the anterior chamber and vitreous. In cases where patients with uveitis experience no relapses for 6 to 12 months, IFN-α is generally tapered down and eventually discontinued [94, 96].

The most common side effect of the drug is flu-like symptoms (90%), which typically resolve within the first few weeks after starting therapy. Nonsteroidal anti-inflammatory drugs, such as paracetamol, can often alleviate these symptoms. Interestingly, the occurrence of flu-like symptoms is considered a positive indicator of IFN therapy efficacy, whereas their absence may suggest the presence of pre-existing or newly developed anti-IFN autoantibodies [57, 97]. Other adverse effects include injection site redness, mild leucopenia, fibromyalgia, depression, hair loss, thrombocytopenia, nausea, vomiting, diarrhea, headache, increase in liver enzyme levels, weight loss, aggressiveness, psychosis, fever, psoriasis, fatigue, loss of appetite, nausea and myalgia arthralgia, alopecia, gastrointestinal disturbances, transient paresthesia, and various central nervous system symptoms, such as epilepsy. A rare but severe adverse event is the development of anti-DNA and anti-thyroid antibodies (occurring in less than 1% of treated patients), which may occasionally lead to the exacerbation of pre-existing autoimmune diseases or the onset of new autoimmune conditions [13, 57, 93]. Also, IFN retinopathy has been reported in patients treated for uveitis [98].

5.7 Janus kinase inhibitors

Janus kinase (JAK) inhibitors represent a novel class of immunomodulatory agents, including tofacitinib, baricitinib, peficitinib, filgotinib, and upadacitinib. Among these, tofacitinib has been successfully incorporated into the treatment of BD. Additionally, the JAK-1 selective inhibitor upadacitinib has been approved for the management of rheumatoid arthritis, psoriatic arthritis, ankylosing spondylitis, and inflammatory bowel disease. Although the use of upadacitinib for treating BD has not been previously reported, two case reports have demonstrated its efficacy in managing uveitis [99].

5.8 Vitreoretinal surgery

Medical therapy remains the cornerstone of management in BU. However, considering its recurrent nature and potential vision-threatening complications, surgical intervention might be necessary in the selected cases.

Retinal vasculitis in BU can lead to ischemia-driven neovascularization, predisposing to recurrent vitreous hemorrhages. Persistent or recurrent hemorrhage causing severe visual impairment despite medical therapy warrants vitreoretinal surgery in these cases. Chronic inflammation can lead to ERM formation, inducing macular traction and distortion, compromising visual acuity. A vitreoretinal surgery, including pars plana vitrectomy with membrane peeling, may be necessary in these cases to alleviate traction and improve retinal architecture. Ischemia and chronic inflammation may result in tractional retinal detachment due to fibrovascular proliferation. Additionally, in some cases, BU-associated retinal vasculitis may predispose to rhegmatogenous retinal detachment. Pars plana vitrectomy, with or without additional scleral buckling and endotamponade, is necessary to reattach the retina in these patients. In addition, a macular hole is another indication for vitreoretinal surgery in patients with BU [100, 101].

Performing vitreoretinal surgery in BD presents unique challenges due to the inflammatory nature of the disease. Several factors must be addressed to optimize surgical outcomes. As BD is characterized by episodic inflammation, and intraocular surgery can trigger disease exacerbation. Adequate immunosuppressive therapy should be optimized preoperatively to minimize postoperative inflammation. Collaboration with rheumatologists or immunologists is essential to ensure systemic disease control. Intraoperative considerations involve employing a minimally traumatic technique to minimize surgical stress and inflammation. In cases of BD that underwent surgical treatment, inflammation may worsen postoperatively, necessitating additional aggressive steroid or immunosuppressive therapy to manage the increased inflammatory response and prevent further complications [100, 102].

5.9 Panretinal photocoagulation

Panretinal photocoagulation (PRP) may be necessary to manage neovascularization secondary to chronic ischemic retinal vasculitis in patients with BU. Optic disc and/or retinal neovascularization resulting from retinal ischemia can be confirmed using FA, which reveals areas of retinal non-perfusion. In these cases, PRP is an effective treatment modality, addressing the ischemic retina and controlling neovascular growth by inducing retinal scarring, thereby reducing the risk of severe complications such as vitreous hemorrhage or retinal detachment [103].

Adjunctive therapy with anti-vascular endothelial growth factor (anti-VEGF) agents may be employed to manage acute neovascularization. These agents stabilize the neovascularization and help prevent further vascular leakage or hemorrhage. However, the long-term efficacy and role of anti-VEGF therapy in BU remain uncertain, particularly due to the chronic inflammatory nature of the disease and the potential recurrence of retinal vasculitis.

Considerations for PRP treatment in BU focus on timing the procedure appropriately to minimize the risk of exacerbating underlying inflammation. One of the most critical aspects of management is ensuring that inflammation is well-controlled before proceeding with PRP. Active retinal vasculitis or significant inflammation can worsen following PRP, leading to further complications.

Therefore, an aggressive approach to inflammation control—using corticosteroids or immunosuppressive agents—is often necessary before initiating PRP to minimize these risks [100, 104].

Overall, while PRP remains a cornerstone in treating ischemic retinal complications in BU, careful patient selection, precise timing, and diligent management of inflammation are essential to achieving optimal outcomes and preventing further retinal damage.

In summary, conventional immunosuppressive agents such as azathioprine, cyclosporine A, and corticosteroids, as well as biologic agents like INF-α and anti-TNF-α, have proven effective in the treatment of BU. However, these agents may be insufficient for controlling inflammation in severe cases, or their side effects could limit their use. The efficacy of anti-interleukin-1 agents, such as anakinra and canakinumab, has been demonstrated in case reports and small retrospective studies of patients with BU, with or without ocular involvement [80]. Other potential treatments currently under investigation, aside from anti-TNF-α agents, include interleukin inhibitors such as IL-1, IL-17, IL-12/23, as well as rituximab and JAK inhibitors. Gevokizumab, an IL-1 inhibitor, and secukinumab, an IL-17 inhibitor, have shown promising clinical responses in reducing ocular disease severity in cases of refractory and chronic uveitis. In contrast, IL-12/23 inhibitors (like ustekinumab) and JAK inhibitors, which have demonstrated early promising results in controlling noninfectious uveitis, are still too early in their research to confirm their long-term efficacy for anti-inflammatory control. Alternatively, rituximab may be considered for ocular BD, though studies suggest it is not superior to older conventional therapies [19].

6. Conclusions

Behçet's disease is a complex condition that demands a multidisciplinary approach. The prompt and effective treatment of uveitis attacks, ensuring rapid resolution of intraocular inflammation, is essential to preventing vision loss in patients with BD. Destructive and recurrent attacks particularly those involving the posterior segment and retina, increase the risk of permanent alterations in the sensory retina, resulting in irreversible vision loss. The management strategy focuses on promptly suppressing inflammation during acute attacks and preventing recurrence. To achieve this, both local and systemic approaches are utilized, including immunosuppressive agents, corticosteroids, and biologic therapies. The effectiveness and safety of interferon-alpha, infliximab, and adalimumab for treating uveitis in BU have been established through recent controlled trials, extensive clinical cohorts, and long-term follow-up studies. Recent studies have highlighted the positive impact of new biologic therapies, specific receptor antagonists such as tocilizumab and secukinumab, as well as JAK inhibitors, on overall disease control and the improvement of quality of life in patients with BU. However, there is no doubt that extensive, multicenter, and well-structured studies are essential to enhance our understanding of these new treatment modalities.

Conflict of interest

The author(s) declare no conflict of interest.

Author details

Seher Köksaldı
Department of Ophthalmology, Agri Ibrahim Cecen University, Faculty of Medicine, Agri, Turkey

*Address all correspondence to: seherkoksaldi@gmail.com

References

[1] Duszynski RJ, Topczewski J, LeClair EE. Divergent requirements for fibroblast growth factor signaling in zebrafish maxillary barbel and caudal fin regeneration. Development, Growth & Differentiation. 2013;**55**(2):282-300

[2] Dai L, Huang F, Jiang Q, Guo S, Tan S, Su G, et al. Sensitive optical coherence tomography angiography parameters detecting retinal vascular changes in Behçet's uveitis. Photodiagnosis and Photodynamic Therapy. 2024;**49**:104353

[3] Yang P, Fang W, Meng Q, Ren Y, Xing L, Kijlstra A. Clinical features of Chinese patients with Behçet's disease. Ophthalmology. 2008;**115**(2):312-8.e4

[4] Mesquida M, Llorenç V, Fontenla JR, Navarro MJ, Adán A. Use of ultra-wide-field retinal imaging in the management of active Behçet retinal vasculitis. Retina. 2014;**34**(10):2121-2127

[5] Criteria for diagnosis of Behçet's disease. International Study Group for Behçet's disease. Lancet. 1990;**335**(8697):1078-1080

[6] International Team for the Revision of the International Criteria for Behçet's Disease (ITR-ICBD). The international criteria for Behçet's disease (ICBD): A collaborative study of 27 countries on the sensitivity and specificity of the new criteria. Journal of the European Academy of Dermatology and Venereology. 2014;**28**(3):338-347

[7] McNally TW, Damato EM, Murray PI, Denniston AK, Barry RJ. An update on the use of biologic therapies in the management of uveitis in Behçet's disease: A comprehensive review. Orphanet Journal of Rare Diseases. 2017;**12**(1):130

[8] Direskeneli H. Behçet's disease: Infectious aetiology, new autoantigens, and HLA-B51. Annals of the Rheumatic Diseases. 2001;**60**(11):996-1002

[9] Savey L, Resche-Rigon M, Wechsler B, Comarmond C, Piette JC, Cacoub P, et al. Ethnicity and association with disease manifestations and mortality in Behçet's disease. Orphanet Journal of Rare Diseases. 2014;**9**:42

[10] Koné-Paut I, Geisler I, Wechsler B, Ozen S, Ozdogan H, Rozenbaum M, et al. Familial aggregation in Behçet's disease: High frequency in siblings and parents of pediatric probands. The Journal of Pediatrics. 1999;**135**(1):89-93

[11] Kaur M, Yip K. The current and novel imaging modalities for ocular vasculitis in Behçet's disease: A review. Cureus. 2024;**16**(9):e69528

[12] Ksiaa I, Abroug N, Kechida M, Zina S, Jelliti B, Khochtali S, et al. Eye and Behçet's disease. Journal Français d'Ophtalmologie. 2019;**42**(6):626-641

[13] Hazirolan D, Stübiger N, Pleyer U. Light on the horizont: Biologicals in Behçet uveitis. Acta Ophthalmologica. 2013;**91**(4):297-306

[14] Hatemi G, Seyahi E, Fresko I, Talarico R, Hamuryudan V. Behçet's syndrome: A critical digest of the 2014-2015 literature. Clinical and Experimental Rheumatology. 2015;**33** (6 Suppl. 94):S3-S14

[15] Tugal-Tutkun I, Gupta V, Cunningham ET. Differential diagnosis of Behçet uveitis. Ocular Immunology and Inflammation. 2013;**21**(5):337-350

[16] Namba K, Goto H, Kaburaki T, Kitaichi N, Mizuki N, Asukata Y,

et al. A major review: Current aspects of ocular Behçet's disease in Japan. Ocular Immunology and Inflammation. 2015;**23**(Suppl. 1):S1-S23

[17] Cunningham ET Jr, Tugal-Tutkun I, Khairallah M, Okada AA, Bodaghi B, Zierhut M. Behçet Uveitis. Ocular Immunology and Inflammation. 2017;**25**(1):2-6

[18] Tugal-Tutkun I, Onal S, Altan-Yaycioglu R, Huseyin Altunbas H, Urgancioglu M. Uveitis in Behçet disease: An analysis of 880 patients. American Journal of Ophthalmology. 2004;**138**(3):373-380

[19] Khieu C, Chanthan D. Novel approach to Behçet's disease in the era of biologic agents. Current Opinion in Ophthalmology. 2023;**34**(6):535-542

[20] Ozyazgan Y, Ucar D, Hatemi G, Yazici Y. Ocular involvement of Behçet's syndrome: A comprehensive review. Clinical Reviews in Allergy and Immunology. 2015;**49**(3):298-306

[21] Markomichelakis NN, Aissopou EK, Maselos S, Tugal-Tutkun I, Sfikakis PP. Biologic treatment options for retinal neovascularization in Behçet's disease. Ocular Immunology and Inflammation. 2019;**27**(1):51-57

[22] Morton LT, Situnayake D, Wallace GR. Genetics of Behçet's disease. Current Opinion in Rheumatology. 2016;**28**(1):39-44

[23] Keino H. Evaluation of disease activity in uveoretinitis associated with Behçet's disease. Immunological Medicine. 2021;**44**(2):86-97

[24] Tugal-Tutkun I, Onal S, Stanford M, Akman M, Twisk JWR, Boers M, et al. An algorithm for the diagnosis of Behçet disease uveitis in adults. Ocular Immunology and Inflammation. 2021;**29**(6):1154-1163

[25] Tugal-Tutkun I. Imaging in the diagnosis and management of Behçet disease. International Ophthalmology Clinics. 2012;**52**(4):183-190

[26] Tugal-Tutkun I, Cingü K, Kir N, Yeniad B, Urgancioglu M, Gül A. Use of laser flare-cell photometry to quantify intraocular inflammation in patients with Behçet uveitis. Graefe's Archive for Clinical and Experimental Ophthalmology. 2008;**246**(8):1169-1177

[27] Yu HG, Kim MJ, Oh FS. Fluorescein angiography and visual acuity in active uveitis with Behçet disease. Ocular Immunology and Inflammation. 2009;**17**(1):41-46

[28] Tugal-Tutkun I, Onal S, Altan-Yaycioglu R, Kir N, Urgancioglu M. Neovascularization of the optic disc in Behçet's disease. Japanese Journal of Ophthalmology. 2006;**50**(3):256-265

[29] Zając H, Turno-Kręcicka A. Ocular manifestations of Behçet's disease: An update on diagnostic challenges and disease management. Journal of Clinical Medicine. 2021;**10**(21):5174

[30] Tugal-Tutkun I, Ozdal PC, Oray M, Onal S. Review for diagnostics of the year: Multimodal imaging in Behçet uveitis. Ocular Immunology and Inflammation. 2017;**25**(1):7-19

[31] Oray M, Onal S, Bayraktar S, Izgi B, Tugal-Tutkun I. Nonglaucomatous localized retinal nerve fiber layer defects in Behçet uveitis. American Journal of Ophthalmology. 2015;**159**(3):475-81.e1

[32] Khairallah M, Abroug N, Khochtali S, Mahmoud A, Jelliti B, Coscas G, et al. Optical coherence tomography angiography in

patients with Behçet uveitis. Retina. 2017;**37**(9):1678-1691

[33] Mesquida M, Molins B, Llorenç V, Hernández MV, Espinosa G, Dick AD, et al. Current and future treatments for Behçet's uveitis: Road to remission. International Ophthalmology. 2014;**34**(2):365-381

[34] Saadoun D, Wechsler B, Terrada C, Hajage D, Le Thi HD, Resche-Rigon M, et al. Azathioprine in severe uveitis of Behçet's disease. Arthritis Care & Research (Hoboken). 2010;**62**(12):1733-1738

[35] Tanaka T, Suzuki J, Yamakawa N, Usui M. Steroid sensitivity and postoperative course of seven patients with Behçet's disease. Ophthalmic Research. 2000;**32**(1):41-43

[36] Li B, Chi K, Li H, Wang J, Zheng Y. Optimizing Behçet uveitis management: A review of personalized immunosuppressive strategies. Medical Science Monitor. 2024;**30**:e943240

[37] Lescrauwaet B, Miserocchi E, Thurau S, Bodaghi B, Duchateau L, Verstraeten T, et al. Association between visual function response and reduction of inflammation in noninfectious uveitis of the posterior segment. Investigative Ophthalmology & Visual Science. 2017;**58**(9):3555-3562

[38] Herbort CP Jr, Tugal-Tutkun I, Neri P, Pavésio C, Onal S, LeHoang P. Failure to integrate quantitative measurement methods of ocular inflammation hampers clinical practice and trials on new therapies for posterior uveitis. Journal of Ocular Pharmacology and Therapeutics. 2017;**33**(4):263-277

[39] Hatemi G, Silman A, Bang D, Bodaghi B, Chamberlain AM, Gul A, et al. EULAR recommendations for the management of Behçet disease. Annals of the Rheumatic Diseases. 2008;**67**(12):1656-1662

[40] Shugaiv E, Tüzün E, Mutlu M, Kiyat-Atamer A, Kurtuncu M, Akman-Demir G. Mycophenolate mofetil as a novel immunosuppressant in the treatment of neuro-Behçet's disease with parenchymal involvement: Presentation of four cases. Clinical and Experimental Rheumatology. 2011;**29**(4 Suppl. 67): S64-S67

[41] Zierhut M, Abu El-Asrar AM, Bodaghi B, Tugal-Tutkun I. Therapy of ocular Behçet disease. Ocular Immunology and Inflammation. 2014;**22**(1):64-76

[42] Jap A, Chee SP. Immunosuppressive therapy for ocular diseases. Current Opinion in Ophthalmology. 2008;**19**(6):535-540

[43] Deuter CM, Kötter I, Wallace GR, Murray PI, Stübiger N, Zierhut M. Behçet's disease: Ocular effects and treatment. Progress in Retinal and Eye Research. 2008;**27**(1):111-136

[44] Hemady RK, Chan AS, Nguyen AT. Immunosuppressive agents and nonsteroidal anti-inflammatory drugs for ocular immune and inflammatory disorders. Ophthalmology Clinics of North America. 2005;**18**(4):511-528 vi

[45] Davatchi F, Sadeghi Abdollahi B, Shams H, Shahram F, Nadji A, Chams-Davatchi C, et al. Combination of pulse cyclophosphamide and azathioprine in ocular manifestations of Behçet's disease: Longitudinal study of up to 10 years. International Journal of Rheumatic Diseases. 2014;**17**(4):444-452

[46] Yates PA, Michelson JB. Behçet disease. International Ophthalmology Clinics. 2006;**46**(2):209-233

[47] Hatemi G, Christensen R, Bang D, Bodaghi B, Celik AF, Fortune F, et al. 2018 update of the EULAR recommendations for the management of Behçet's syndrome. Annals of the Rheumatic Diseases. 2018;**77**(6):808-818

[48] BenEzra D, Cohen E, Chajek T, Friedman G, Pizanti S, de Courten C, et al. Evaluation of conventional therapy versus cyclosporine A in Behçet's syndrome. Transplantation Proceedings. 1988;**20**(3 Suppl. 4):136-143

[49] Kato Y, Numaga J, Kato S, Kaburaki T, Kawashima H, Fujino Y. Central nervous system symptoms in a population of Behçet's disease patients with refractory uveitis treated with cyclosporine A. Clinical & Experimental Ophthalmology. 2001;**29**(5):335-336

[50] Sakane T, Mochizuki M, Inaba G, Masuda K. A phase II study of FK506 (tacrolimus) on refractory uveitis associated with Behçet's disease and allied conditions. Ryūmachi. 1995;**35**(5):802-813

[51] Kilmartin DJ, Forrester JV, Dick AD. Tacrolimus (FK506) in failed cyclosporin A therapy in endogenous posterior uveitis. Ocular Immunology and Inflammation. 1998;**6**(2):101-109

[52] Yurdakul S, Mat C, Tüzün Y, Ozyazgan Y, Hamuryudan V, Uysal O, et al. A double-blind trial of colchicine in Behçet's syndrome. Arthritis and Rheumatism. 2001;**44**(11):2686-2692

[53] Feldmann M, Brennan FM, Foxwell BM, Maini RN. The role of TNF alpha and IL-1 in rheumatoid arthritis. Current Directions in Autoimmunity. 2001;**3**:188-199

[54] Murphy CC, Greiner K, Plskova J, Duncan L, Frost A, Isaacs JD, et al. Neutralizing tumor necrosis factor activity leads to remission in patients with refractory noninfectious posterior uveitis. Archives of Ophthalmology. 2004;**122**(6):845-851

[55] Elezoglou AV, Sfikakis PP, Vaiopoulos G, Kapsimali V, Kaklamanis PG. Serum levels of soluble TNF-alpha receptor-II (P75), circulating gammadelta T-cells and Adamantiades-Behçet's disease activity. Advances in Experimental Medicine and Biology. 2003;**528**:261-265

[56] Sfikakis PP, Kaklamanis PH, Elezoglou A, Katsilambros N, Theodossiadis PG, Papaefthimiou S, et al. Infliximab for recurrent, sight-threatening ocular inflammation in Adamantiades-Behçet disease. Annals of Internal Medicine. 2004;**140**(5):404-406

[57] Kötter I, Günaydin I, Zierhut M, Stübiger N. The use of interferon alpha in Behçet disease: Review of the literature. Seminars in Arthritis and Rheumatism. 2004;**33**(5):320-335

[58] Yamada Y, Sugita S, Tanaka H, Kamoi K, Takase H, Mochizuki M. Timing of recurrent uveitis in patients with Behçet's disease receiving infliximab treatment. The British Journal of Ophthalmology. 2011;**95**(2):205-208

[59] Tugal-Tutkun I, Mudun A, Urgancioglu M, Kamali S, Kasapoglu E, Inanc M, et al. Efficacy of infliximab in the treatment of uveitis that is resistant to treatment with the combination of azathioprine, cyclosporine, and corticosteroids in Behçet's disease: An open-label trial. Arthritis and Rheumatism. 2005;**52**(8):2478-2484

[60] Robertson LP, Hickling P. Treatment of recalcitrant orogenital ulceration of Behçet's syndrome with infliximab. Rheumatology (Oxford, England). 2001;**40**(4):473-474

[61] Goossens PH, Verburg RJ, Breedveld FC. Remission of Behçet's syndrome with tumour necrosis factor alpha blocking therapy. Annals of the Rheumatic Diseases. 2001;**60**(6):637

[62] Levy-Clarke G, Jabs DA, Read RW, Rosenbaum JT, Vitale A, Van Gelder RN. Expert panel recommendations for the use of anti–tumor necrosis factor biologic agents in patients with ocular inflammatory disorders. Ophthalmology. 2014;**121**(3):785-796 e3

[63] Mushtaq B, Saeed T, Situnayake RD, Murray PI. Adalimumab for sight-threatening uveitis in Behçet's disease. Eye (London, England). 2007;**21**(6):824-825

[64] Interlandi E, Leccese P, Olivieri I, Latanza L. Adalimumab for treatment of severe Behçet's uveitis: A retrospective long-term follow-up study. Clinical and Experimental Rheumatology. 2014;**32**(4 Suppl. 84):S58-S62

[65] Church LD, McDermott MF. Canakinumab, a fully-human mAb against IL-1beta for the potential treatment of inflammatory disorders. Current Opinion in Molecular Therapeutics. 2009;**11**(1):81-89

[66] Yoshimura T, Sonoda KH, Ohguro N, Ohsugi Y, Ishibashi T, Cua DJ, et al. Involvement of Th17 cells and the effect of anti-IL-6 therapy in autoimmune uveitis. Rheumatology (Oxford, England). 2009;**48**(4):347-354

[67] Hamzaoui K, Hamzaoui A, Guemira F, Bessioud M, Hamza M, Ayed K. Cytokine profile in Behçet's disease patients. Relationship with disease activity. Scandinavian Journal of Rheumatology. 2002;**31**(4):205-210

[68] Deroux A, Chiquet C, Bouillet L. Tocilizumab in severe and refractory Behçet's disease: Four cases and literature review. Seminars in Arthritis and Rheumatism. 2016;**45**(6):733-737

[69] Hirano T, Ohguro N, Hohki S, Hagihara K, Shima Y, Narazaki M, et al. A case of Behçet's disease treated with a humanized anti-interleukin-6 receptor antibody, tocilizumab. Modern Rheumatology. 2012;**22**(2):298-302

[70] Shapiro LS, Farrell J, Borhani HA. Tocilizumab treatment for neuro-Behçet's disease, the first report. Clinical Neurology and Neurosurgery. 2012;**114**(3):297-298

[71] Papo M, Bielefeld P, Vallet H, Seve P, Wechsler B, Cacoub P, et al. Tocilizumab in severe and refractory non-infectious uveitis. Clinical and Experimental Rheumatology. 2014;**32**(4 Suppl. 84): S75-S79

[72] Emmi G, Silvestri E, Squatrito D, Emmi L, Cantarini L, Prisco D. Tocilizumab-induced exacerbation of mucosal ulcers in a patient with multi-refractory Behçet′s disease. Seminars in Arthritis and Rheumatism. 2016;**46**(1):e1-e2

[73] Cantarini L, Lopalco G, Vitale A, Coladonato L, Rigante D, Lucherini OM, et al. Paradoxical mucocutaneous flare in a case of Behçet's disease treated with tocilizumab. Clinical Rheumatology. 2015;**34**(6):1141-1143

[74] Teoh SC, Sharma S, Hogan A, Lee R, Ramanan AV, Dick AD. Tailoring biological treatment: Anakinra treatment of posterior uveitis associated with the CINCA syndrome. The British Journal of Ophthalmology. 2007;**91**(2):263-264

[75] Cantarini L, Vitale A, Scalini P, Dinarello CA, Rigante D, Franceschini R, et al. Anakinra treatment in drug-resistant Behçet's disease: A case

series. Clinical Rheumatology. 2015;**34**(7):1293-1301

[76] Emmi G, Talarico R, Lopalco G, Cimaz R, Cantini F, Viapiana O, et al. Efficacy and safety profile of anti-interleukin-1 treatment in Behçet's disease: A multicenter retrospective study. Clinical Rheumatology. 2016;**35**(5):1281-1286

[77] Geiler J, McDermott MF. Gevokizumab, an anti-IL-1β mAb for the potential treatment of type 1 and 2 diabetes, rheumatoid arthritis and cardiovascular disease. Current Opinion in Molecular Therapeutics. 2010;**12**(6):755-769

[78] Gül A, Tugal-Tutkun I, Dinarello CA, Reznikov L, Esen BA, Mirza A, et al. Interleukin-1β-regulating antibody XOMA 052 (gevokizumab) in the treatment of acute exacerbations of resistant uveitis of Behçet's disease: An open-label pilot study. Annals of the Rheumatic Diseases. 2012;**71**(4):563-566

[79] Tugal-Tutkun IM, Kadayifcilar SM, Khairallah MM, Lee SCMP, Ozdal P, Özyazgan Y, et al. Safety and efficacy of gevokizumab in patients with Behçet's disease uveitis: Results of an exploratory phase 2 study. Ocular Immunology and Inflammation. 2017;**25**(1):62-70

[80] Tugal-Tutkun I, Pavesio C, De Cordoue A, Bernard-Poenaru O, Gül A. Use of gevokizumab in patients with Behçet's disease uveitis: An international, randomized, double-masked, placebo-controlled study and open-label extension study. Ocular Immunology and Inflammation. 2018;**26**(7):1023-1033

[81] Sanford M, McKeage K. Secukinumab: First global approval. Drugs. 2015;**75**(3):329-338

[82] Sota J, Rigante D, Lopalco G, Frediani B, Franceschini R, Galeazzi M, et al. Biological therapies for the treatment of Behçet's disease-related uveitis beyond TNF-alpha blockade: A narrative review. Rheumatology International. 2018;**38**(1):25-35

[83] Dick AD, Tugal-Tutkun I, Foster S, Zierhut M, Melissa Liew SH, Bezlyak V, et al. Secukinumab in the treatment of noninfectious uveitis: Results of three randomized, controlled clinical trials. Ophthalmology. 2013;**120**(4):777-787

[84] Baerveldt EM, Kappen JH, Thio HB, van Laar JA, van Hagen PM, Prens EP. Successful long-term triple disease control by ustekinumab in a patient with Behçet's disease, psoriasis and hidradenitis suppurativa. Annals of the Rheumatic Diseases. 2013;**72**(4):626-627

[85] Buggage RR, Levy-Clarke G, Sen HN, Ursea R, Srivastava SK, Suhler EB, et al. A double-masked, randomized study to investigate the safety and efficacy of daclizumab to treat the ocular complications related to Behçet's disease. Ocular Immunology and Inflammation. 2007;**15**(2):63-70

[86] Evereklioglu C, Er H, Türköz Y, Cekmen M. Serum levels of TNF-alpha, sIL-2R, IL-6, and IL-8 are increased and associated with elevated lipid peroxidation in patients with Behçet's disease. Mediators of Inflammation. 2002;**11**(2):87-93

[87] Kempen JH, Gangaputra S, Daniel E, Levy-Clarke GA, Nussenblatt RB, Rosenbaum JT, et al. Long-term risk of malignancy among patients treated with immunosuppressive agents for ocular inflammation: A critical assessment of the evidence. American Journal of Ophthalmology. 2008;**146**(6):802-12.e1

[88] Sadreddini S, Noshad H, Molaeefard M, Noshad R. Treatment of retinal vasculitis in Behçet's disease

with rituximab. Modern Rheumatology. 2008;**18**(3):306-308

[89] Davatchi F, Shams H, Rezaipoor M, Sadeghi-Abdollahi B, Shahram F, Nadji A, et al. Rituximab in intractable ocular lesions of Behçet's disease; randomized single-blind control study (pilot study). International Journal of Rheumatic Diseases. 2010;**13**(3):246-252

[90] Ruck T, Bittner S, Wiendl H, Meuth SG. Alemtuzumab in multiple sclerosis: Mechanism of action and beyond. International Journal of Molecular Sciences. 2015;**16**(7):16414-16439

[91] Lockwood CM, Hale G, Waldman H, Jayne DR. Remission induction in Behçet's disease following lymphocyte depletion by the anti-CD52 antibody CAMPATH 1-H. Rheumatology (Oxford, England). 2003;**42**(12):1539-1544

[92] Mohammad AJ, Smith RM, Chow YW, Chaudhry AN, Jayne DR. Alemtuzumab as remission induction therapy in Behçet disease: A 20-year experience. The Journal of Rheumatology. 2015;**42**(10):1906-1913

[93] Deuter C, Stübiger N, Zierhut M. Interferon-α therapy in noninfectious uveitis. Developments in Ophthalmology. 2012;**51**:90-97

[94] Tugal-Tutkun I, Güney-Tefekli E, Urgancioglu M. Results of interferon-alfa therapy in patients with Behçet uveitis. Graefe's Archive for Clinical and Experimental Ophthalmology. 2006;**244**(12):1692-1695

[95] Onal S, Kazokoglu H, Koc A, Akman M, Bavbek T, Direskeneli H, et al. Long-term efficacy and safety of low-dose and dose-escalating interferon alfa-2a therapy in refractory Behçet uveitis. Archives of Ophthalmology. 2011;**129**(3):288-294

[96] Kötter I, Eckstein AK, Stübiger N, Zierhut M. Treatment of ocular symptoms of Behçet's disease with interferon alpha 2a: A pilot study. The British Journal of Ophthalmology. 1998;**82**(5):488-494

[97] Deuter CM, Kötter I, Günaydin I, Stübiger N, Doycheva DG, Zierhut M. Efficacy and tolerability of interferon alpha treatment in patients with chronic cystoid macular oedema due to non-infectious uveitis. The British Journal of Ophthalmology. 2009;**93**(7):906-913

[98] Plskova J, Greiner K, Forrester JV. Interferon-alpha as an effective treatment for noninfectious posterior uveitis and panuveitis. American Journal of Ophthalmology. 2007;**144**(1):55-61

[99] Tao T, He D, Peng X, Huang Z, Su W. Successful remission with Upadacitinib in two patients with anti-TNF-refractory macular edema associated with Behçet's uveitis. Ocular Immunology and Inflammation. 2024;**32**(8):1897-1900

[100] Ksiaa I, Abroug N, Kechida M, Zina S, Jelliti B, Khochtali S, et al. Eye and Behçet's disease. Journal Français d'Ophtalmologie. 2019;**42**(4):e133-ee46

[101] Gasparian SA, Barrett D, Sierpina D, Chalam KV. Successful repair of combined tractional and rhegmatogenous retinal detachment with pars plana vitrectomy without scleral buckle in severe Behçet's disease. Journal of Surgical Case Reports. 2020;**2020**(11):rjaa468

[102] Khalil H, Gendy HAE, Raafat HA, Haroun HE, Gheita TA, Bakir HM. The effectiveness of pre- and postoperative infliximab in controlling Behçet's disease posterior uveitis in patients undergoing

vitrectomy: A preliminary study. Journal of Ophthalmology. 2017;**2017**:8168369

[103] Atmaca LS, Batioğlu F, Idil A. Retinal and disc neovascularization in Behçet's disease and efficacy of laser photocoagulation. Graefe's Archive for Clinical and Experimental Ophthalmology. 1996;**234**(2):94-99

[104] Stuebiger N, Koetter I, Zierhut M. Complete regression of retinal neovascularization after therapy with interferon alfa in Behçet's disease. The British Journal of Ophthalmology. 2000;**84**(12):1437-1438

Section 3

Surgical and Global Perspectives

Chapter 6

Glaucoma Drainage Implants for Uveitic Glaucoma

Gianluca Besozzi, Michele Santoro, Flavio Cassano, Milena L'Abbate and Maria Carmela Costa

Abstract

Uveitic glaucoma (UG) is a complex secondary glaucoma caused by intraocular inflammation that disrupts aqueous humor drainage, leading to increased intraocular pressure (IOP) and potential vision loss. While medical therapy is the first-line treatment, glaucoma drainage implants (GDIs) become essential when pharmacologic management fails. Common GDIs, including the Ahmed Glaucoma Valve (AGV), Baerveldt Glaucoma Implant (BGI), and Molteno implant, play a critical role, particularly in cases with chronic inflammation. Successful GDI surgery requires meticulous preoperative planning, with strict inflammation control being paramount. Device selection is crucial, with valved implants (e.g., Ahmed Glaucoma Valve) often preferred for better IOP regulation and lower hypotony risk. Surgical techniques must consider conjunctival handling, incision approach, and implant positioning to optimize outcomes. Postoperative management focuses on inflammation control, IOP monitoring, and wound healing. Potential complications, such as hypotony, a hypertensive phase, tube occlusion, erosion, and infection, necessitate prompt intervention. Advancements in surgical approaches, including novel biomaterials, microshunts, minimally invasive glaucoma surgery (MIGS), and drug-eluting implants, aim to enhance safety and efficacy. GDIs remain a cornerstone in the management of uveitic glaucoma, necessitating individualized treatment strategies and continued innovation.

Keywords: uveitic glaucoma, glaucoma drainage implants, GDI, ahmed glaucoma valve, baerveldt glaucoma implant, molteno implant, glaucoma surgery, microinvasive glaucoma surgery, MIGS

1. Introduction

Uveitic glaucoma is a complex and challenging condition that frequently manifests as a secondary form of glaucoma associated with intraocular inflammation. It arises in the context of uveitis, which involves inflammation of the uveal tract (iris, ciliary body, and choroid) and can disrupt normal aqueous humor drainage and/or increase its production, ultimately leading to elevated intraocular pressure (IOP). Left untreated, this condition can result in irreversible optic nerve damage and vision loss [1, 2].

The underlying inflammatory processes of uveitic glaucoma significantly affect both the trabecular meshwork (TM) and the conventional outflow pathways, making its management particularly difficult. While medical therapies aimed at reducing IOP and controlling inflammation remain the first-line treatment, surgical intervention becomes essential in cases where medical management fails or the glaucoma is refractory. Traditional treatments, including topical medications, laser procedures, and filtering surgeries, may carry increased risks in the context of uveitis. Consequently, glaucoma drainage implants (GDIs) have become a critical option for managing these patients [3].

GDIs, such as the Ahmed Glaucoma Valve, Baerveldt Glaucoma Implant, and Molteno implant, are indispensable in managing uveitic glaucoma, especially in cases with chronic inflammation or complex disease presentations where other surgical modalities may not be viable. These devices provide a reliable method to lower IOP and achieve long-term control in patients with this challenging condition.

2. Uveitic glaucoma: An overview

2.1 Pathophysiology of uveitic glaucoma

The pathophysiology of uveitic glaucoma revolves around the imbalance between aqueous humor production and its drainage from the eye. Inflammation, whether from acute or chronic uveitis and corticosteroid use, often leads to structural changes in the anterior segment of the eye that affect both the trabecular meshwork (TM) and the uveoscleral outflow pathway. Furthermore, neovascularization of the iris (NVI) and subsequent neovascular glaucoma (NVG) can occur in chronic uveitis due to ischemic retinal vasculitis, chronic inflammation, and vascular endothelial growth factor (VEGF) upregulation.

These changes include:

- *Inflammatory cell infiltration*: The infiltration of inflammatory cells (lymphocytes, neutrophils) into the trabecular meshwork leads to obstruction and fibrosis, significantly impeding aqueous outflow. This is especially prominent in chronic cases of uveitis, where ongoing inflammation causes permanent damage to the outflow pathways [4].

- *Increased aqueous humor production*: In some forms of uveitis, such as iritis or anterior uveitis, increased production of aqueous humor from the ciliary body is a major contributor to elevated IOP. Chronic inflammation in the ciliary body can lead to further dysregulation of fluid dynamics within the eye [5].

- *Synechiae and iris bombe*: These conditions, caused by the adhesion of the iris to the lens or corneal endothelium, are common in uveitis and can obstruct the angle, leading to angle-closure glaucoma.

- *Extracellular matrix deposition*: Corticosteroids affect the function of the trabecular meshwork by modifying cellular activity, which results in decreased aqueous humor outflow. This reduction is primarily caused by the accumulation of extracellular matrix and the consequent dysfunction of the trabecular meshwork [6].

- *Neovascularization of the angle (NVA)*: Abnormal blood vessels grow along the trabecular meshwork and iris. This leads to the formation of a fibrovascular membrane, which can contract and cause peripheral anterior synechiae (PAS), resulting in angle closure. The obstruction of the trabecular meshwork impairs aqueous humor outflow, increasing intraocular pressure (IOP).

These alterations in aqueous humor dynamics make uveitic glaucoma difficult to manage and increase the likelihood of surgical intervention when medical therapies fail.

2.2 Corticosteroids in uveitis

Corticosteroids remain a cornerstone of uveitis treatment, effectively reducing inflammation, preventing tissue damage, and preserving visual function. However, careful monitoring is necessary due to the risk of corticosteroid-induced ocular hypertension [6]. To minimize long-term corticosteroid use and its associated complications, steroid-sparing agents are frequently employed, including immunosuppressive agents as well as biologic therapies. Corticosteroids play a dual role in uveitic glaucoma, as they are essential for controlling inflammation while simultaneously contributing to IOP elevation and glaucoma progression [6].

2.3 Risk factors for uveitic glaucoma

Several factors increase the likelihood of developing uveitic glaucoma:

- *Systemic autoimmune and inflammatory conditions*: Conditions, such as rheumatoid arthritis, sarcoidosis, Behçet's disease, and systemic lupus erythematosus (SLE), are strongly associated with uveitic glaucoma.

- *Chronic and recurrent episodes of uveitis*: These episodes predispose individuals to increased risks of secondary glaucoma.

- *Age and gender*: Younger patients are at a higher risk for developing uveitic glaucoma, particularly those with juvenile idiopathic arthritis-associated uveitis. In addition, male patients are more frequently affected by Behçet's disease, which commonly leads to uveitic glaucoma.

- *History of ocular trauma*: Prior eye injury may increase the likelihood of developing uveitic glaucoma due to scarring or synechiae formation.

3. Selection criteria for glaucoma drainage implant surgery in uveitic glaucoma

The decision to proceed with GDI surgery in uveitic glaucoma requires a thorough evaluation of multiple factors, aiming to balance the potential benefits against the risks [2]. Surgical intervention is generally indicated when medical therapy and laser procedures fail to adequately control intraocular pressure (IOP) or when there is evidence of progressive optic nerve damage despite treatment. Key considerations include:

1. *Failure of prior treatments*:

    - *Medical therapy*: Surgery is warranted if maximal tolerated medical therapy fails to control IOP or if the patient exhibits intolerance to medications, such as steroids or systemic immunosuppressive agents commonly used in uveitis management [7].

    - *Laser procedures*: Laser trabeculoplasty and cyclophotocoagulation, though sometimes effective for temporary relief, often fail to provide sustained IOP reduction in the presence of active or chronic uveitis [8].

    - *Trabeculectomy failure*: In uveitic glaucoma, trabeculectomy is associated with a higher risk of failure due to fibrosis and inflammation. GDIs are often preferred, particularly in eyes with significant scarring or neovascular glaucoma [1].

2. *Type and severity of uveitis*:

    - *Active inflammation*: It is crucial to control active inflammation before surgery, as ongoing inflammation increases the likelihood of fibrosis, poor wound healing, and surgical failure [9].

    - *Chronic or recurrent uveitis*: Persistent inflammatory mediators in chronic uveitis can promote scar tissue formation around the implant, potentially compromising its efficacy [10].

    - *Specific uveitic entities*: Different types of uveitis (e.g., anterior, intermediate, posterior) present varying surgical challenges. Anterior uveitis may directly impact anterior segment surgery, while posterior uveitis increases the risk of complications, such as tube occlusion or hypotony [11].

3. *Intraocular pressure considerations*:

    - *Uncontrolled IOP*: GDI surgery is typically indicated when IOP remains uncontrolled, despite maximal therapy [7].

    - *Progressive optic nerve damage*: Even if the IOP is not exceedingly high, progressive visual field loss or optic nerve damage necessitates surgical intervention [7].

    - *Target IOP*: Due to the unpredictable nature of inflammation, uveitic glaucoma patients often require a personalized IOP target that balances sufficient IOP reduction with the risk of hypotony.

4. *Presence of concomitant ocular conditions*:

    - *Cataracts*: In patients with cataracts, combined phacoemulsification with GDI implantation may improve both IOP control and visual outcomes [12].

    - *Corneal pathologies*: Corneal scarring or keratopathy can influence surgical timing and technique [1].

- *Keratoprosthesis*: For patients requiring keratoprosthesis (KPro) due to severe corneal disease, GDIs are often implanted in the pars plana to achieve effective IOP control [13].

5. *Patient compliance and accessibility*:

- *Treatment adherence*: Successful outcomes depend on the patient's ability to adhere to a rigorous postoperative care regimen.

- *Access to care*: Proximity to medical facilities for regular follow-up is a critical factor, as uveitic glaucoma management often requires close monitoring.

4. Surgical techniques and special considerations in uveitic glaucoma

GDI surgery in uveitic glaucoma necessitates a tailored approach, encompassing both the general principles of GDI implantation and the specific challenges arising from intraocular inflammation [1]. Uveitic glaucoma is a complex condition often requiring a nuanced surgical strategy.

4.1 Device selection

Several different types of GDIs are available, each with unique characteristics (**Table 1**). The most commonly used implants include:

- *Ahmed Glaucoma Valve (AGV)* (**Figures 1** and **2**): This is a valved implant designed to regulate the flow of aqueous humor and minimize the risk of excessive drainage and subsequent hypotony [1]. The AGV is particularly advantageous in cases of uveitic glaucoma, where its ability to manage inflammation is beneficial [2]. It also functions well in eyes with chronic inflammation or fibrosis [14]. The valve is designed to restrict outflow when the IOP is less than 8–12 mmHg. The Ahmed Glaucoma Valve (AGV) is available in various models and sizes, including single and double plates, with polypropylene or silicone plate materials.

- *Baerveldt Glaucoma Implant (BGI)* (**Figure 3**): This is a non-valved implant characterized by a larger surface area designed to provide more controlled drainage [9]. Due to its larger size, the BGI is typically implanted under the rectus

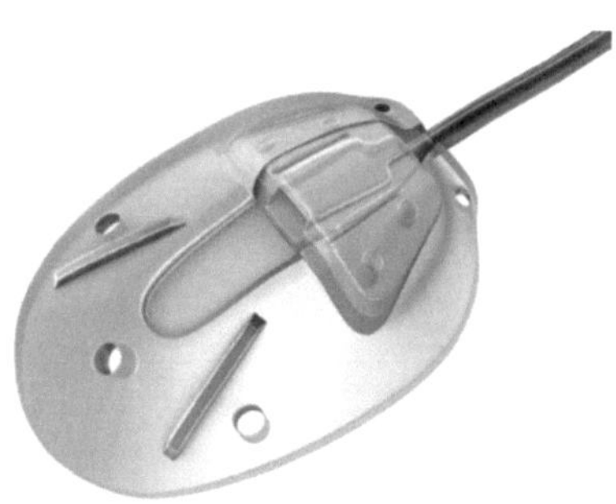

Figure 1.
AGV.

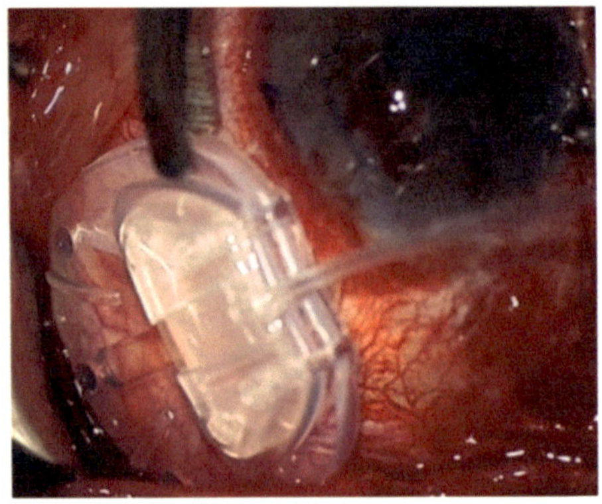

Figure 2.
AGV placement during surgery.

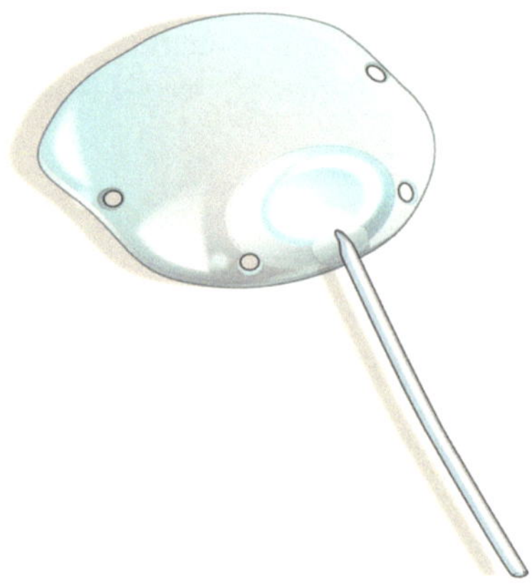

Figure 3.
BGI.

muscles, which can make the surgery more challenging [10]. It has proven effective in managing advanced glaucoma and in cases where previous surgeries have failed [14]. The BGI's lack of a valve makes it more susceptible to early hypotony and may require a temporary tube ligation to control initial flow.

- *Molteno implant*: One of the earliest types of drainage devices, the Molteno implant is particularly useful in managing complex, refractory glaucoma cases [11]. Its larger drainage surface facilitates effective drainage, but its non-valved design makes it prone to hypotony, necessitating close postoperative monitoring and tube ligation (Video 1 http://bit.ly/4bZEhSl) [1].

- *Aurolab Aqueous Drainage Implant (AADI)*: The AADI is a non-valved device manufactured in India that serves as a cost-effective alternative [12]. It is similar in design to the Baerveldt and requires tube ligation [12].

- *Newer implant systems*: Advances in GDI technology have introduced new materials and designs aimed at improving patient outcomes. These include the use of more biocompatible materials, such as silicone and polyethylene, which aim to reduce the foreign body response that can contribute to inflammation and device failure. Integrated valves and porous structures in some devices are designed to better regulate aqueous flow and minimize the risk of complications [15].

Each implant type has its indications based on the specific needs of the patient, including IOP levels, severity of inflammation, and the likelihood of scarring. Choosing the appropriate implant requires careful preoperative assessment and surgical planning.

- *Valved vs. non-valved implants* (**Table 1**): The selection between valved (e.g., Ahmed Glaucoma Valve—AGV) and non-valved (e.g., Baerveldt Glaucoma Implant—BGI, Molteno implant) GDIs is crucial and depends on the patient's particular condition and the surgeon's discretion [1]. Valved devices, like the AGV, are often preferred due to their capacity to offer better immediate intraocular pressure (IOP) control and diminish the risk of postoperative hypotony, which is particularly important in patients with unstable uveitis [2]. The AGV's valve mechanism restricts aqueous outflow when IOP drops below 8–12 mmHg, reducing the likelihood of hypotony [2]. Non-valved devices such as the BGI, while potentially providing better long-term IOP control through a larger drainage area, require a temporary ligature or stent to prevent early hypotony [2]. The choice often hinges on the need for immediate IOP reduction versus long-term stability.

- *Specific preference for AGV*: The Ahmed Glaucoma Valve (AGV) is frequently favored in uveitic glaucoma cases due to its valved mechanism. This valve is designed to restrict outflow when the IOP is less than 8 mmHg [9]. This is critical for reducing the risk of early hypotony, a complication that can be particularly problematic in the context of uveitic eyes with compromised tissue integrity [1]. The valve's ability to limit overfiltration is key in these cases.

- *Implant size and material*: Larger plate sizes may enhance IOP reduction due to an increased surface area available for aqueous outflow, but they also come with a heightened risk of hypotony [7]. *The correlation between larger plate size and lower*

Device	Characteristics	Advantages	Limitations
Ahmed Glaucoma Valve (AGV)	Valved implant minimizes excessive drainage and hypotony. Available in various models and materials (polypropylene, silicone).	Effective in uveitic glaucoma and eyes with chronic inflammation or fibrosis. Reduced early hypotony risk.	May not provide as extensive long-term IOP control as non-valved devices.
Baerveldt Glaucoma Implant (BGI)	Non-valved implant, large drainage surface.	Effective for advanced glaucoma and failed surgeries; provides long-term IOP control.	Prone to hypotony; requires close monitoring tube ligation; more challenging surgery due to larger size.
Molteno Implant	Non-valved, large drainage surface.	Useful in managing complex, refractory glaucoma.	Prone to hypotony; requires close monitoring and tube ligation

Table 1.
Valved vs. non-valved glaucoma implants.

IOP is observed up to a certain extent, without necessarily improving the overall success rate [8]. The material composition of the implant may influence its biocompatibility and the ensuing inflammatory response [12]. For instance, *silicone end plates are typically less inflammatory than polypropylene* [16]. The selection of implant material also affects the tissue reaction and bleb encapsulation [17].

A retrospective study compared Ahmed and Baerveldt implants in 137 eyes of patients with uveitic glaucoma. The results indicated that the Baerveldt implant achieved a greater reduction in intraocular pressure (IOP) (60.3 vs. 44.5% with the Ahmed implant). However, the Baerveldt implant was associated with a higher complication rate (51.4 vs. 20.9% with the Ahmed implant), including hypotony [18].

A retrospective study by Valenzuela et al. evaluated the long-term efficacy of the Ahmed GDI in patients with refractory uveitic glaucoma. The cumulative probability of success, according to the Kaplan-Meier analysis, was 65% at 84 months [19].

A retrospective study by Vuori assessed the efficacy of the Molteno implant in patients with uveitic glaucoma. The study reported qualified success rates of 97, 93, 90, and 85% at 1, 2, 3, and 4 years, respectively. Success was defined as achieving an intraocular pressure (IOP) within the target range with or without adjunctive medication [20].

4.2 Surgical techniques and special considerations

- *Surgical timing*: In cases of uveitic glaucoma, *it is often necessary to control the inflammation*, prior to considering any surgical intervention to achieve better surgical outcomes [15]. Surgical success is compromised by the presence of uncontrolled inflammation [21].

- *Conjunctival management*: *Fluid-assisted dissection* is recommended to avoid buttonholing of the conjunctiva, especially in scarred tissue [3]. A *peritomy* at the 9 to 12 o'clock or 12 to 3 o'clock positions is favored, depending on the eye being operated upon [3]. Subconjunctival injection of *4% lidocaine with adrenaline* facilitates both hemostasis and tissue separation from the sclera [3]. Meticulous conjunctival dissection is crucial to *prevent holes or tears* [3].

- *Incision technique*: A scleral tunnel approach is often preferred over a direct incision to reduce the risk of tube exposure and erosion [22]. This technique involves creating a partial-thickness scleral tunnel to pass the tube, ensuring that the tube does not directly impinge upon the conjunctiva [22].

- *Implant placement*

In cases where the superotemporal quadrant is not viable due to conjunctival scarring or previous surgical interventions, alternative quadrants may be considered. These include the superonasal, inferotemporal, and inferonasal quadrants [3]. The inferotemporal quadrant, for example, is often selected to reduce the likelihood of diplopia in patients who maintain good binocular vision [23]. On the other hand, placement in the nasal quadrants requires meticulous attention to avoid optic nerve damage, particularly if the GDI plate is positioned too posteriorly [3].

In eyes containing silicone oil, the implant may be placed in either the superior or inferior quadrants depending on the clinical scenario [9]. For patients with a history of scleral buckle surgery, the choice of quadrant becomes more complex. The quadrant

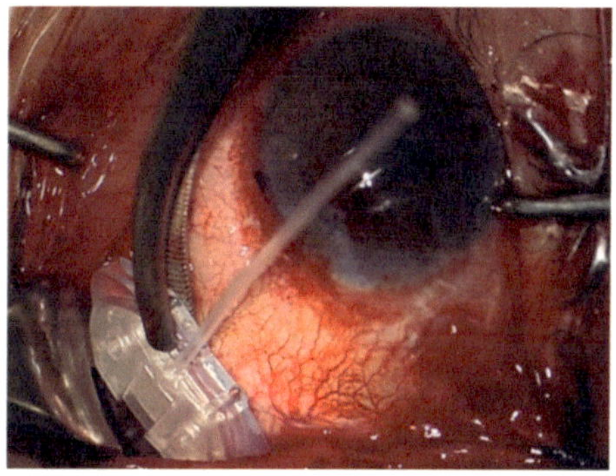

Figure 4.
GDD implantation in the superotemporal quadrant.

containing the buckle is generally avoided due to the difficulties in securing the implant [3]. In cases where conjunctival scarring is extensive, alternative strategies may include the use of pediatric-sized implants or trimming an adult implant to fit the available space [3]. These adjustments are crucial for ensuring that the device remains functional while minimizing the risks of complications in anatomically challenging eyes.

4.3 Tube insertion into the anterior chamber

The precise placement of the tube within the anterior chamber is a critical factor in determining the success of GDI surgery. Proper positioning and secure fixation of the tube significantly influence the procedure's efficacy, safety, and long-term outcomes.

The intra-anterior chamber length of the tube should ideally measure approximately 2 mm, as this length ensures sufficient aqueous drainage while minimizing the risk of complications such as corneal endothelial cell loss [1]. To further reduce this risk, the tube must be inserted with the bevel facing upwards (**Figure 5**), a technique that mitigates iris occlusion and helps preserve endothelial integrity [2]. The insertion site is ideally positioned as far as possible from the corneal endothelial surface. In

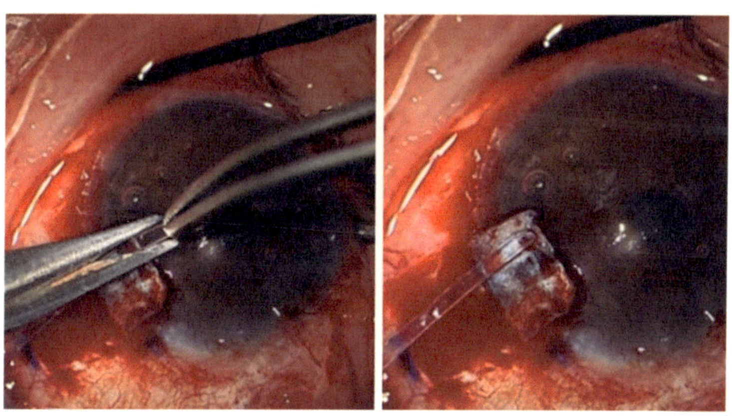

Figure 5.
Tube cut beveled up.

such cases, minimizing contact between the tube and the graft reduces the likelihood of endothelial damage [23]. Eyes with a deep anterior chamber allow the tube to be positioned near the iris, maintaining adequate distance from the cornea. Conversely, in phakic patients with a shallow anterior chamber, GDI implantation is generally contraindicated due to the heightened risk of corneal touch [14].

The technique used for tube insertion is equally important. The needle tract method is commonly employed, wherein a 23G needle is used to create a track approximately 4 mm posterior to the limbus. The needle is initially directed vertically beneath the episclera before being aligned parallel to the iris [7]. During this process, viscoelastic substances are injected to prevent sudden decompression and reduce the risk of postoperative hypotony [7]. Once the track is prepared, the tube is inserted using atraumatic forceps or an inserter [24].

Secure fixation of the tube to the sclera is essential to prevent migration or extrusion. The tube is typically secured with 9-0 nylon sutures to minimize micromovements, ensuring stability over time [1].

For tube coverage, various graft materials, including scleral, corneal, or pericardial tissue, are used to protect the tube near the limbus. These grafts are fixed in place with 9-0 or 10-0 monofilament nylon sutures, preventing tube exposure and erosion [1]. Alternative surgical techniques, such as the graft-free method or the Sherwood slit technique, may also be employed to address specific challenges. The graft-free technique involves creating a scleral tunnel for tube passage, while the Sherwood slit technique incorporates a small cut in the tube to facilitate fluid escape and reduce hypotony [6, 14].

4.4 Use of adjunctive medications

- *Mitomycin C (MMC)*: Intraoperative application of MMC can help reduce postoperative fibrosis but must be used with caution due to the risk of hypotony [25]. While some studies have shown positive results using MMC, its use in uveitic glaucoma might increase inflammation, necessitating a more conservative approach.

- *Steroids*: Intra- and postoperative corticosteroids are crucial for controlling inflammation [5]. They can be given topically, orally, or as intravitreal injections depending on the severity of the inflammatory process.

- *Anti-VEGF agents*: In neovascular glaucoma associated with uveitis, intravitreal injections of bevacizumab may be used to reduce neovascularization before or during GDI surgery.

4.5 Trabeculectomy vs. traditional GDIs

Trabeculectomy, although a standard surgical procedure for glaucoma, has significant limitations in uveitic glaucoma due to chronic inflammation associated with uveitis, which can compromise surgical success [26].

Uveitis is characterized by persistent intraocular inflammation. Elevated levels of transforming growth factor-beta (TGF-β) and other growth factors in the aqueous humor promote fibroblast activation, collagen contraction, and scarring, increasing the risk of bleb fibrosis and surgical failure [26].

Due to the risks associated with trabeculectomy, glaucoma drainage devices (GDIs) are often preferred in uveitic glaucoma. GDIs provide an alternative aqueous outflow pathway, reducing reliance on the filtration bleb and lowering the risk of fibrosis-related failure. In uveitic glaucoma with significant IOP fluctuations, tube shunts demonstrate better outcomes compared to trabeculectomy. GDIs remain a viable surgical option when trabeculectomy fails [26].

GDIs offer a more reliable surgical alternative but require meticulous inflammation management to ensure long-term success.

5. Management of GDI surgery-related complications in uveitic glaucoma

Patients with uveitic glaucoma undergoing GDI surgery are at an increased risk of complications due to the underlying inflammation and altered tissue responses [27]. Early detection and prompt management of complications are crucial for successful outcomes:

5.1 Early postoperative hypotony

Early postoperative hypotony, a potential complication following GDI surgery, arises from various mechanisms and requires prompt identification and management. Excessive aqueous outflow is a common cause, particularly in cases involving non-valved devices that lack a mechanism to restrict drainage. This uncontrolled outflow can lead to dangerously low IOP. Additionally, ciliary body shutdown, often due to inflammation or surgical trauma, may reduce aqueous production, compounding hypotony.

Management of early hypotony includes several strategies aimed at stabilizing IOP and addressing underlying causes. For non-valved devices, tube ligation using a temporary dissolvable ligature, such as a Vicryl suture, is frequently employed to regulate outflow during the initial postoperative weeks. The ligature dissolves gradually over 3 to 5 weeks, allowing controlled aqueous flow as healing progresses.

Topical steroids play a critical role in reducing inflammation and addressing ciliary body dysfunction, while cycloplegic agents, such as atropine 1%, stabilize the blood-ocular barrier and mitigate the risk of aqueous misdirection [28]. For persistent hypotony, the injection of viscoelastic material into the anterior chamber can temporarily elevate IOP, providing both diagnostic and therapeutic intervention. This approach also aids in detecting potential leaks, allowing for targeted corrective measures.

By addressing the specific causes of hypotony and implementing appropriate interventions, early postoperative complications can be minimized, improving outcomes for patients undergoing GDI implantation.

5.2 Late postoperative hypotony

5.2.1 Late postoperative hypotony: Causes and management

Late postoperative hypotony, which can develop months or even years after GDI surgery, is often the result of several underlying mechanisms. One of the primary causes is chronic overfiltration, which typically arises when a mature bleb forms, especially with non-valved implants. As the bleb matures, it may become excessively permeable, leading to prolonged aqueous outflow and low IOP. Additionally, persistent ciliary body dysfunction, which may stem from inflammation, aging, or other factors, further contributes to reduced aqueous production, exacerbating hypotony. In some cases, the development of a cyclodialysis cleft, a complication associated with GDIs, can lead to chronic hypotony. Bleb leaks are another contributing factor, potentially resulting in fluid loss that further reduces IOP.

In the context of uveitic glaucoma, chronic inflammation can lead to prolonged ciliary body dysfunction and bleb fibrosis, increasing the risk of hypotony.

Management of late hypotony generally involves a combination of conservative and surgical approaches. The use of increased topical steroid drops or systemic steroids is often the first line of treatment to reduce inflammation and help restore normal aqueous production. When combined with atropine drops, which help to prevent ciliary body shutdown, this regimen may provide effective control over hypotony. In cases where conservative management fails, viscoelastic injections into the anterior chamber can help assess the chamber's ability to retain fluid and can provide valuable insight into whether leakage or surgical revision is necessary. If these measures are insufficient, surgical interventions such as plate reduction (in Baerveldt implants), tube ligation, or, in more severe cases, implant removal may be required to address persistent hypotony and restore IOP control.

Timely and effective management of late postoperative hypotony is essential to prevent vision loss and ensure long-term success following GDI implantation.

5.3 Hypertensive phase

The hypertensive phase typically occurs around 6 weeks after GDI surgery and is characterized by an increase in IOP. The primary cause of this phase is the encapsulation of the GDI plate, which leads to reduced aqueous outflow and a subsequent rise in IOP.

Management of the hypertensive phase generally begins with medical treatment. Additionally, digital massage to the bleb may improve aqueous outflow and alleviate the elevated pressure. In more resistant cases, where medical management alone is insufficient, surgical revision may be necessary. This can include needling of the bleb with the application of antimetabolites to break down the encapsulating tissue, or the removal of the tube ligature to restore normal aqueous flow. Early recognition and appropriate intervention are crucial.

5.4 Tube occlusion

Tube occlusion is a potential complication that can arise following GDI surgery, where various factors contribute to the blockage of the tube. Common causes of tube occlusion include blood clots, vitreous, fibrin, or inflammatory debris, all of which can impede the normal flow of aqueous humor through the tube [27]. The presence of these obstructions can lead to elevated IOP and compromise the effectiveness of the drainage system.

Management of tube occlusion typically involves addressing the blockage through tube irrigation, which may help clear the obstruction and restore normal fluid flow. In more severe cases, surgical revision may be necessary to remove the blockage and ensure the continued function of the implant. For vitreous occlusion, a vitrectomy procedure may be required to remove the vitreous body or any debris obstructing the tube. Timely intervention is critical to prevent complications associated with uncontrolled IOP and to maintain the long-term success of the surgical outcome.

5.5 Tube erosion and exposure

Tube erosion and exposure represent significant complications following GDI surgery. Erosion of the conjunctiva or Tenon's capsule can result in the tube becoming exposed, creating a direct pathway for infection and further complications [29]. This exposure increases the risk of endophthalmitis or other infectious processes that can jeopardize the success of the surgery.

The management of tube erosion typically involves surgical repair aimed at covering the exposed portion of the tube to reduce the risk of infection. This is often achieved by using a scleral patch graft, corneal graft, or amniotic membrane, which provides a protective barrier over the exposed tube and promotes healing of the surrounding tissue [30, 29].

5.6 Infection (endophthalmitis)

Infection, particularly endophthalmitis, poses a significant risk following GDI surgery, and this risk may be heightened in patients with uveitis due to their underlying inflammatory condition. The immunosuppressed status associated with uveitis, as well as the potential for compromised tissue integrity, increases the likelihood of postoperative infection [31].

Prompt recognition and early intervention are crucial to managing endophthalmitis effectively. Intravitreal antibiotics are typically administered to address the infection rapidly. In severe cases where infection does not resolve with medical treatment, explantation of the GDI may be necessary to prevent further complications and preserve the integrity of the eye [31].

5.7 Strabismus and ptosis

Strabismus and ptosis can occur as complications following GDI placement, often resulting from the positioning of the device or the surgical intervention itself. Misalignment of the eye muscles, which leads to strabismus, and drooping of the eyelid, or ptosis, may arise as a consequence of the pressure exerted by the GDI or the surgical manipulation during the procedure [32].

The management of these complications typically requires surgical intervention. For strabismus, corrective surgery may be necessary to realign the eye muscles, while ptosis may require specific repair procedures to lift the eyelid and restore proper function.

5.8 Bleb-related complications

Bleb-related complications are common following GDI surgery and can significantly impact the success of the procedure. One such complication is the fibrous encapsulation of the bleb, which can lead to reduced aqueous outflow, ultimately increasing IOP. Another issue is bleb leaks, which may result in hypotony and heighten the risk of infection.

Managing these complications typically involves bleb needling, often combined with the use of antimetabolites to promote appropriate healing and prevent further scarring. In cases where needling is not sufficient, surgical revision may be necessary.

6. Emerging techniques and innovations

Research in glaucoma surgery continues to evolve, with several promising innovations that may enhance the safety and efficacy of GDI in uveitic glaucoma:

- *Newer materials*:
- *Microshunts*:
    - o InnFocus MicroShunt**:** This device utilizes a biocompatible material and shunts aqueous humor to a subconjunctival space, with promising results in early studies. The device is implanted through an *ab externo* approach with minimal tissue dissection.
- *Minimally invasive glaucoma surgery (MIGS)*:
    - o iStent (**Figure 6**): The iStent inject device, designed to improve aqueous flow through Schlemm's canal, might help in lowering IOP in mild-to-moderate glaucoma cases. It has a self-trephining tip and is designed to be inserted through a clear corneal incision.
    - o *XEN Gel Stent*: This device, composed of porcine gelatin cross-linked with glutaraldehyde, is inserted through a 27-gauge needle, creating a new drainage pathway to the subconjunctival space and may be useful for uveitic glaucoma patients.
    - o *Drug-eluting implants*:

6.1 MIGS vs. traditional GDIs

Minimally invasive glaucoma surgery (MIGS) and traditional GDI represent two distinct approaches to glaucoma management, each with specific indications, advantages, and limitations (**Table 2**).

MIGS involves an *ab interno* approach with gonioscopic assistance, characterized by lower invasiveness and conjunctival sparing. The recovery time is generally rapid, and the procedure is largely independent of bleb formation. MIGS tends to achieve a moderate reduction in IOP while maintaining a high safety profile. The risk of complications is minimal, with reported adverse events including transient IOP spikes, intraoperative blood reflux from Schlemm's canal, stent malposition, and obstruction.

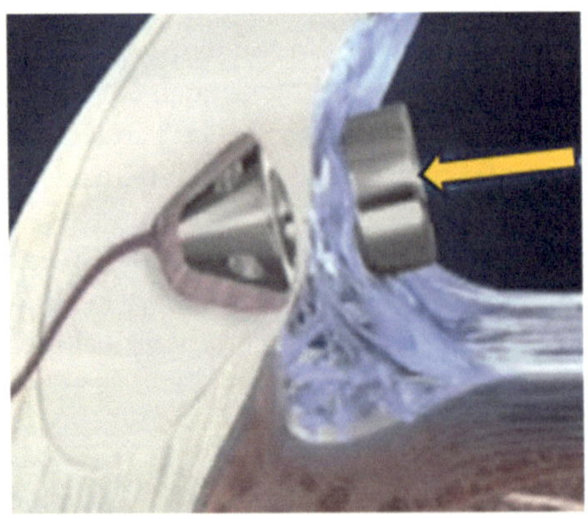

Figure 6.
iStent.

	MIGS	Traditional GDI
Invasiveness	Lower Conjunctival sparing	More invasive May compromise conjunctiva
Recovery time	Rapid	Slower
Common complications	Transient IOP spikes, blood reflux, stent malposition, obstruction	Hypotony, outflow obstruction, conjunctival erosion, implant exposure, tube migration, diplopia, corneal decompensation, endophthalmitis
Indications	Mild-to-moderate primary open-angle glaucoma, secondary open-angle glaucomas, coexisting cataract	Refractory glaucomas, secondary glaucomas uncontrolled with maximal medical therapy, high-risk patients for filtration surgery failure
Contraindications	Advanced glaucoma, angle-closure glaucomas, previous glaucoma surgery, low IOP target needs	Angle-closure glaucomas

Table 2.
MIGS vs. traditional GDI.

MIGS is primarily indicated for primary open-angle glaucoma and secondary open-angle glaucomas, such as pigmentary and pseudoexfoliative glaucoma, particularly in cases of mild-to-moderate disease and when cataract surgery is also planned. However, it is contraindicated in primary and secondary angle-closure glaucomas, advanced glaucomas, patients with a history of previous glaucoma surgery, and cases requiring a very low target IOP [33].

In contrast, traditional GDI procedures are more invasive but have been demonstrated to effectively lower IOP and preserve vision. These devices are primarily indicated for refractory glaucomas or cases unlikely to respond to conventional filtration surgery. They are also used in secondary glaucomas that remain uncontrolled despite maximal tolerated medical therapy, as well as in patients at high risk of filtration surgery failure. GDI is also indicated in patients at high risk of filtration surgery failure, those with conjunctival scarring, and in cases of neovascular glaucoma.

However, GDI procedures are associated with a higher incidence of complications.

In conclusion, MIGS should be considered a first-line surgical option for uveitic glaucoma in cases where moderate IOP reduction is sufficient, and preserving the conjunctiva is paramount. Its minimally invasive nature and favorable safety profile make it particularly advantageous for patients with mild-to-moderate disease. However, for advanced or refractory UG, traditional GDI procedures remain indispensable due to their superior ability to achieve and maintain significant IOP reduction.

6.2 Innovative technologies

Magnetically actuated implants (eyeWatch) (**Figure** 7): a promising, non-invasive approach to adjusting IOP after glaucoma surgery. A new GDI with an integrated magnetic microvalve allows external modulation of hydrodynamic resistance, enabling precise IOP control. This technology is suitable for patients with glaucoma from mild to severe [34].

Self-Adjustable Glaucoma Drainage Device (SAGDD): It is a novel implant for glaucoma treatment designed to maintain IOP within a desired range. SAGDDs

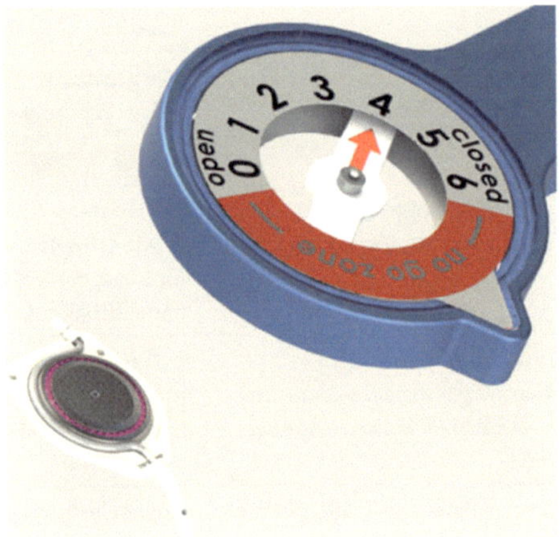

Figure 7.
eyeWatch.

dynamically modulate fluidic resistance, preventing postoperative hypotony and long-term hypertension. It includes a flexible membrane that deforms in response to pressure changes, adjusting flow resistance and stabilizing IOP. Inspired by the Starling resistor, the SAGDD features a simple and potentially cost-effective design. Unlike other devices, such as the eyeWatch, the SAGDD self-regulates without the need for human intervention [35].

7. Selective laser trabeculoplasty (SLT) and cyclophotocoagulation (CPC) in uveitic glaucoma

SLT is a non-invasive laser procedure that targets pigmented trabecular meshwork cells to improve aqueous humor outflow and lower IOP. It is performed in an outpatient setting, is repeatable, and can reduce IOP by 20–30%. However, its efficacy is variable, particularly in cases with severe trabecular damage or synechial closure. SLT may also exacerbate ocular inflammation and cause transient IOP spikes, posing risks for some patients [36]. In particular, patients with uveitic glaucoma are at risk of intraocular inflammation flare-ups after SLT, as the pro-inflammatory nature of the procedure may trigger a recurrence of uveitis. Additionally, patients with elevated preoperative IOP may be more susceptible to post-SLT IOP spikes [36]. CPC reduces IOP by ablating the ciliary body to decrease aqueous humor production. It is effective for refractory UG cases and can be performed under local anesthesia. While it provides substantial IOP reduction, CPC may worsen intraocular inflammation and carries a risk of inducing hypotony. The response to CPC is unpredictable [37].

8. Postoperative care

Postoperative care following GDI surgery in uveitic glaucoma is crucial for long-term success [5]. The patient should undergo frequent follow-up visits, particularly in the initial postoperative months, to monitor for potential complications. Strategies include:

8.1 Monitoring inflammation and wound healing

The most critical aspect of postoperative care in uveitic glaucoma is the management of inflammation. Topical corticosteroids and cycloplegics are frequently used to reduce inflammation and to prevent excessive fibrosis and maintain bleb function [5]. However, systemic immunosuppressive agents and oral steroids might be required for patients with active inflammation due to underlying autoimmune disease.

8.2 IOP monitoring

Close monitoring of IOP is essential, especially during the early postoperative period and around the time of tube ligature removal (for non-valved devices) or during the hypertensive phase (for valved devices) [5].

8.3 Wound management

Proper conjunctival healing is critical to prevent tube erosion or exposure [22]. Scleral or amniotic membrane grafts may be used to reinforce compromised conjunctival tissue [38].

8.4 Ensuring tube patency

It is essential to monitor tube patency regularly. This can be done through slit-lamp examination, gonioscopy, and advanced imaging techniques, such as *anterior segment optical coherence tomography (AS-OCT)*, which allows for detailed assessment of the tube and surrounding tissues without invasive procedures. In case of tube occlusion, a sterile irrigation procedure might be necessary.

9. Juvenile idiopathic arthritis (JIA) management

JIA is a chronic inflammatory condition that can cause severe ocular complications, particularly uveitis. Among the most challenging consequences of JIA-associated uveitis are band keratopathy and aphakia, which present significant difficulties in the context of uveitic glaucoma and the surgical management involving GDI.

Band keratopathy, caused by calcium deposition in the superficial cornea, promoted by chronic inflammation leads to corneal opacity, visual impairment, and ocular discomfort. This condition complicates surgical visualization during GDI implantation. Management typically involves chelation therapy with ethylenediaminetetraacetic acid (EDTA) to dissolve calcium deposits. For deeper deposits, phototherapeutic keratectomy (PTK) with an excimer laser may be required, while severe cases with extensive scarring might necessitate corneal transplantation.

Aphakia often follows complicated cataract extraction, particularly in the setting of uveitic glaucoma. It poses significant challenges, including an increased risk of posterior segment complications, such as cystoid macular edema and hypotony. Inadequate capsular support further complicates intraocular lens (IOL) implantation, leading to refractive instability and a higher risk of amblyopia in pediatric patients. In cases where IOL implantation is feasible, scleral-fixated or anterior chamber IOLs may be used, while iris-claw IOLs offer an alternative for patients with adequate iris support. Aphakic contact lenses remain a practical option for younger patients or those at high surgical risk.

The use of GDI is often necessary for IOP control in JIA-related uveitic glaucoma, particularly when medical therapy proves inadequate [39]. Chronic inflammation increases the risk of fibrosis and device occlusion, while aphakic patients are particularly vulnerable to postoperative hypotony. Flow-regulated devices, such as Ahmed valves, are preferred for patients at high risk of hypotony. Intraoperative use of antifibrotic agents like mitomycin C can reduce the risk of peritubular fibrosis [39].

10. Neovascular glaucoma management

Neovascularization of the iris (NVI) and subsequent NVG can occur in chronic uveitis due to ischemic retinal vasculitis, chronic inflammation, and VEGF upregulation. Neovascular glaucoma (NVG) presents additional challenges due to abnormal blood vessel growth stimulated by retinal ischemia.

Some specific types of uveitis associated with NVG include:

Ischemic retinal vasculitis (e.g., Behçet's disease, Eales disease); intermediate and posterior uveitis with retinal ischemia (e.g., Pars planitis, birdshot chorioretinopathy); infectious uveitis (e.g., tuberculosis, cytomegalovirus (CMV) retinitis, syphilis, Herpetic uveitis)—causing occlusive vasculitis and ischemic changes; autoimmune/granulomatous uveitis (e.g., Sarcoidosis, Vogt-Koyanagi-Harada disease)—leading to chronic vascular inflammation and ischemic damage; uveitis associated with systemic vasculitis (e.g., granulomatosis with polyangiitis (PGA), SLE, polyarteritis nodosa) —resulting in small-vessel occlusion and NVG risk.

10.1 Pathophysiology of NVG in uveitis

Chronic inflammation damages the vascular endothelium.

Retinal ischemia increases VEGF expression, leading to neovascularization.

New vessels form on the iris (NVI) and iridocorneal angle, eventually leading to NVG with angle closure and uncontrolled IOP rise.

Management relies on a combination of pharmacologic and laser treatments to control neovascularization and maintain IOP. Anti-vascular endothelial growth factor (anti-VEGF) agents are crucial in inhibiting neovascularization and reducing vascular permeability and decrease intraocular inflammation. Panretinal photocoagulation (PRP) is another essential intervention, reducing retinal ischemia and inducing regression of neovascular tissue. Early and aggressive treatment with both anti-VEGF therapy and PRP is vital to slow disease progression and prevent further complications [40]. In refractory NVG cases, GDIs are an effective surgical option to maintain long-term IOP control while addressing the underlying neovascular pathology [41].

11. Patient education and counseling for uveitic glaucoma

Uveitic glaucoma, caused by intraocular inflammation and elevated intraocular pressure (IOP), presents significant challenges due to its chronic nature and risk of vision loss. Effective education and counseling are essential for improving patient adherence to treatment and quality of life.

Patients need to understand the basics of uveitic glaucoma. Uveitis causes inflammation that blocks fluid drainage, leading to elevated IOP and potential optic nerve damage. It is important to emphasize the chronic nature of the condition, which requires ongoing monitoring even after surgery. Patients should also be aware that vision loss may occur without obvious symptoms, highlighting the need for regular check-ups.

Patients should understand their treatment plan and the role of GDIs in surgery. Medications like anti-inflammatory or IOP-lowering drops help control inflammation and pressure, but they may not be sufficient in advanced cases. For surgical patients, a GDI helps drain fluid and lower IOP. While GDIs reduce IOP in most cases, they do not cure uveitis or restore vision.

Non-adherence is a common issue. To improve compliance, clinicians should provide a clear medication schedule, particularly during the postoperative period. It is important to stress the need for regular follow-up visits and to address barriers like cost or difficulty administering drops by offering solutions, such as affordable generics or caregiver assistance.

Lifestyle changes can complement treatment. Patients should protect their eyes with sunglasses and safety glasses to avoid ultraviolet (UV) light and trauma. A balanced diet and stress-reduction techniques may support overall health. After GDI surgery, patients should avoid heavy lifting, rubbing the eye, and swimming for 4–6 weeks.

Patients should be educated on symptoms like redness, pain, or sudden vision changes, which may signal complications such as infection or changes in IOP. A 24/7 contact number should be provided for immediate assistance.

Chronic conditions like uveitic glaucoma can affect emotional well-being. Clinicians should validate patient concerns and encourage open dialog. Support groups and counseling services can help patients cope with anxiety, particularly those facing progressive vision loss.

Education should be tailored to different groups. For children with JIA-related uveitic glaucoma, involve parents and use age-appropriate tools. For elderly patients, simplify instructions and address comorbidities. For patients with low health literacy, use plain language and confirm understanding.

Providing patients with helpful resources like one-page summaries, medication reminder apps, and visual aids can improve understanding.

12. Conclusion

The management of uveitic glaucoma remains a challenging domain in clinical ophthalmology, necessitating a comprehensive approach that includes careful patient selection, meticulous surgical techniques, and the proactive management of complications. GDIs play a pivotal role in effectively reducing IOP and preserving vision in this complex condition. By combining advancements in implant technology with effective postoperative care and promptly addressing complications, long-term IOP control and prevention of optic nerve damage can be achieved.

The unique challenges posed by uveitis underscore the importance of multidisciplinary approaches and personalized treatment plans tailored to each patient's specific needs. Emerging technologies and ongoing research into fibrosis prevention, implant design, and personalized medicine hold great promise for improving outcomes. Furthermore, long-term studies comparing the efficacy and safety of various GDI types will be instrumental in guiding clinical decision-making.

As our understanding of uveitic glaucoma continues to evolve, integrating innovative techniques with evidence-based practices will be critical in advancing care and enhancing the quality of life for patients affected by this challenging condition.

Author details

Gianluca Besozzi[1*], Michele Santoro[2], Flavio Cassano[2], Milena L'Abbate[3] and Maria Carmela Costa[2]

1 Sacro Cuore di Gesù Hospital, Gallipoli, Italy

2 Vito Fazzi Hospital, Lecce, Italy

3 Department of Ophthalmology, Vito Fazzi Hospital, Lecce, Italy

*Address all correspondence to: gianlucabesozzi@gmail.com

References

[1] Bhartiya S, Ichhpujani P, Gandhi M. The glaucoma treatment paradigm: An overview. In: Glaucoma Drainage Devices: A Practical Illustrated Guide. Singapore: Springer; 2019. pp. 1-5

[2] Pegu J, Purang A, Gandhi M. Indications of glaucoma drainage implant. In: Glaucoma Drainage Devices: A Practical Illustrated Guide. Singapore: Springer; 2019. pp. 7-12

[3] Ichhpujani P. Preparing the patient for the glaucoma drainage device surgery. In: Glaucoma Drainage Devices: A Practical Illustrated Guide. Singapore: Springer; 2019. pp. 19-24

[4] Cela D, Brignole-Baudouin F, Labbé A, Baudouin C. The trabecular meshwork in glaucoma: An inflammatory trabeculopathy? Journal Français d'Ophtalmologie. 2021;**44**(9):e497-e517

[5] Xiao J, Zhao C, Cheng G, Song H, Zhang Y, Zhang M. Multiple cytokine analysis of aqueous humor in uveitis with or without secondary glaucoma. BMC Ophthalmology. 2024;**24**(1):451

[6] Abouzeid H, Sintzoff L. Corticostéroïdes et glaucome [Corticosteroids and glaucoma]. Revue Médicale Suisse. 2023;**19**(820):643-647. French

[7] Sharma B, Gandhi M, Dubey S, Yadava U. Glaucoma drainage devices: Complications and their management. In: Glaucoma Drainage Devices: A Practical Illustrated Guide. Singapore: Springer; 2019. pp. 117-126

[8] Kaushik S, Joshi G. Postoperative care and follow-up of the patient with glaucoma drainage devices. In: Glaucoma Drainage Devices: A Practical Illustrated Guide. Singapore: Springer; 2019. pp. 127-134

[9] Bhartiya S, Gandhi M. Surgical technique of implantation: AGV, limbal variant. In: Glaucoma Drainage Devices: A Practical Illustrated Guide. Singapore: Springer; 2019. pp. 33-45

[10] Albis-Donado OD, Hernandez-Oteyza A. Glaucoma drainage devices in children. In: Glaucoma Drainage Devices: A Practical Illustrated Guide. Singapore: Springer; 2019. pp. 101-107

[11] Barella K, Costa VP. Modifications of surgical techniques in glaucoma drainage devices. In: Glaucoma Drainage Devices: A Practical Illustrated Guide. Singapore: Springer; 2019. pp. 109-116

[12] Singh M, Mitra A. Economic considerations of glaucoma drainage devices. In: Glaucoma Drainage Devices: A Practical Illustrated Guide. Singapore: Springer; 2019. pp. 143-149

[13] Senthil S. Glaucoma drainage devices: Indications. In: Glaucoma Drainage Devices: A Practical Illustrated Guide. Singapore: Springer; 2019. pp. 74-79

[14] Sharma B, Gandhi M, Yadava U. The glaucoma drainage devices: Types and models. In: Glaucoma Drainage Devices: A Practical Illustrated Guide. Singapore: Springer; 2019. pp. 13-18

[15] Patyal S, Kumar S, Dubey S. Combined phacoemulsification and glaucoma drainage devices. In: Glaucoma Drainage Devices: A Practical Illustrated Guide. Singapore: Springer; 2019. pp. 80-85

[16] Shah PR, Agar A, Clement CI. Molteno implants: Surgical technique. In:

Glaucoma Drainage Devices: A Practical Illustrated Guide. Singapore: Springer; 2019. pp. 67-73

[17] Jutley G, Crawley L. Surgical technique for Baerveldt glaucoma devices. In: Glaucoma Drainage Devices: A Practical Illustrated Guide. Singapore: Springer; 2019. pp. 47-57

[18] Sinha S, Ganjei AY, McWatters Z, Lee D, Moster MR, Myers JS, et al. Ahmed versus Baerveldt glaucoma drainage device in uveitic glaucoma: A retrospective comparative study. Journal of Glaucoma. 2020;**29**(9):750-755

[19] Valenzuela F, Oportus MJ, Pérez CI, Mellado F, Cartes C, Villarroel F, et al. Ahmed glaucoma drainage implant surgery in the management of refractory uveitic glaucoma: Long-term follow up. Archivos de la Sociedad Española de Oftalmología. (English Edition). 2018;**93**(9):431-438. English, Spanish

[20] Vuori ML. Molteno aqueous shunt as a primary surgical intervention for uveitic glaucoma: Long-term results. Acta Ophthalmologica. 2010;**88**(1):33-36. DOI: 10.1111/j.1755-3768.2009.01759.x. Epub 2009 Nov 7

[21] Dubey S, Gupta N, Bhoot M, Singh S. Combined surgeries: Glaucoma drainage devices with Boston KPro. In: Glaucoma Drainage Devices: A Practical Illustrated Guide. Singapore: Springer; 2019. pp. 93-100

[22] Lim KS, Allan BDS, Lloyd AW, Khaw PT. Glaucoma drainage devices; past, present, and future. British Journal of Ophthalmology (United Kingdom). 1998;**82**(10):1083-1089

[23] Bhagat P. The ideal glaucoma drainage device: Which one to choose? In: Glaucoma Drainage Devices: A Practical Illustrated Guide. Springer; 2019. pp. 25-32

[24] Ríos-Acosta N, Corredor-Casas S. Histological considerations of glaucoma drainage devices. In: Glaucoma Drainage Devices: A Practical Illustrated Guide. Singapore: Springer; 2019. pp. 135-142

[25] Sheybani A, Dick HB, Ahmed II. Early clinical results of a novel ab interno gel stent for the surgical treatment of open-angle glaucoma. Journal of Glaucoma. 2016;**25**(7):e691-e696

[26] Kwon HJ, YXG K, Tao LW, Lim LL, Martin KR, Green C, et al. Surgical outcomes of trabeculectomy and glaucoma drainage implant for uveitic glaucoma and relationship with uveitis activity. Clinical & Experimental Ophthalmology. 2017;**45**(5):472-480

[27] Khurana M, Sudhir RR, Rishi E, Sakaria P, Vijaya L. Tube obstruction of a nonvalved glaucoma drainage device by a dislocated Soemmering's ring. Journal of Glaucoma. 2021;**30**(8):e372-e374

[28] Gizzi C, Costa G, Servadei R, Abed E, Ning B, Sharma A, et al. A case of malignant glaucoma following insertion of Preserflo™ MicroShunt. European Journal of Ophthalmology. 2022;**32**(4):NP115-NP119. DOI: 10.1177/11206721211003492. Epub 2021 Mar 18

[29] Nardi M, Maglionico MN, Posarelli C, Figus M. Managing Ahmed glaucoma valve tube exposure: Surgical technique. European Journal of Ophthalmology. 2021;**31**(2):778-781

[30] Liu X, Law SK. Autologous partial-thickness scleral flap and donor corneal graft in management of tube erosion of glaucoma drainage device. Journal of Glaucoma. 2019;**28**(4):347-351

[31] Islam YFK, Blake CR, Gibran SK. Management of endophthalmitis related to glaucoma drainage devices:

Review of the literature and our experience. Eye (London, England). 2021;**35**(7):1850-1858

[32] Roizen A, Ela-Dalman N, Velez FG, Coleman AL, Rosenbaum AL. Surgical treatment of strabismus secondary to glaucoma drainage device. Archives of Ophthalmology. 2008;**126**(4):480-486. DOI: 10.1001/archopht.126.4.480

[33] Lavia C, Dallorto L, Maule M, Ceccarelli M, Fea AM. Minimally-invasive glaucoma surgeries (MIGS) for open angle glaucoma: A systematic review and meta-analysis. PLoS One. 2017;**12**(8):e0183142

[34] Pereira ICF, van Mechelen RJS, Wyss HM, et al. Magnetically actuated glaucoma drainage device for regulating intraocular pressure after implantation. Microsystems & Nanoengineering. 2023;**9**:92

[35] Rafiei S, Gerber JM, Bigler S, Stergiopulos N. A new self-adjustable glaucoma valve. Frontiers in Bioengineering and Biotechnology. 2 May 2024;**12**:1383459

[36] Zhou Y, Pruet CM, Fang C, Khanna CL. Selective laser trabeculoplasty in steroid-induced and uveitic glaucoma. Canadian Journal of Ophthalmology. 2022;**57**(4):277-283. DOI: 10.1016/j.jcjo.2021.05.006. Epub 2021 Jun 11

[37] Khodeiry MM, Liu X, Lee RK. Clinical outcomes of slow-coagulation continuous-wave transscleral cyclophotocoagulation laser for treatment of glaucoma. Current Opinion in Ophthalmology. 2022;**33**(3):237-242

[38] Mills RP, Reynolds A, Emond MJ, et al. Long-term survival of Molteno glaucoma drainage devices. Ophthalmology. 1996;**103**(2):299-305

[39] Glandorf K, Rothaus K, Baquet-Walscheid K, Heinz C, Heiligenhaus A. Surgical glaucoma treatment in patients with juvenile idiopathic arthritis-associated uveitis: Results after trabeculectomy or Ahmed glaucoma valve implantation. Ocular Immunology and Inflammation. 2024;**32**(5):636-641

[40] Dumbrăveanu L, Cușnir V, Bobescu D. A review of neovascular glaucoma. Etiopathogenesis and treatment. Romanian Journal of Ophthalmology. 2021;**65**(4):315-329. DOI: 10.22336/rjo.2021.66

[41] Shchomak Z, Cordeiro Sousa D, Leal I, Abegão PL. Surgical treatment of neovascular glaucoma: A systematic review and meta-analysis. Graefe's Archive for Clinical and Experimental Ophthalmology. 2019;**257**(6):1079-1089

Chapter 7

Perspective Chapter: Challenges in Managing Uveitis in Low- to Middle-Income Countries

Tayyaba Gul Malik and Noor Ul Ain

Abstract

Uveitis is inflammation of uveal tissue, including iris, ciliary body, and choroid. Its presentation varies from a mild idiopathic condition to a severe form of uveitis, which can result in loss of vision if left untreated. Anatomically speaking, it is divided into anterior, intermediate, posterior, and panuveitis. Etiologically, there is a long list of agents. However, idiopathic is the most common type. Geographically, developed countries have a prevalence of autoimmune etiology, and low- and middle-income countries are more prone to infectious uveitis. For example, Tuberculosis, Toxoplasmosis, etc. Uveitis is associated with systemic diseases too. Hence, a multidisciplinary approach is mandatory in its management. It requires resources, collaboration, manpower, and diagnostic facilities, which are scarce in LMICs, making uveitis a challenging disease in these areas. Health budgets are already drained in LMICs and budget allocated to the ocular conditions is far from what is actually needed. This is further complicated by the high burden of infectious diseases. There is a scarcity of trained specialists, making coordination among different disciplines a huge challenge with already compromised healthcare. The patients present late when vision salvage becomes extremely difficult. Broadly speaking, national guidelines that are true representative of the affected region are absent, and poor infrastructure, cultural barriers, ignorance, and illiteracy aggravate the situation. It is important to address these issues through a multifaceted approach. Budget allocation for preventable blindness and infectious ocular diseases, innovations in diagnostics, public awareness campaigns, improving access to care, and specialized training can improve the condition. In addition, the use of technology such as teleophthalmology, artificial intelligence, and mobile health can help in bridging the gaps. All-out efforts need to be done at the national and international levels to reduce the burden of uveitis and prevent blindness caused by this debilitating disease.

Keywords: uveitis, tuberculosis, sarcoidosis, panuveitis, choroiditis

1. Introduction

Uveitis is not a single disease entity. It is inflammation of the uveal tissue, but it can be a part of a wide variety of systemic diseases, making diagnosis and treatment a challenge for ophthalmologists. Although anatomically it is divided into anterior,

IntechOpen

intermediate, posterior, and panuveitis, many other classifications are found in literature depending on etiology, systems involved and causative organisms. Many of the uveitis have a characteristic pattern which helps in reaching a diagnosis. However, its versatile nature and multisystem involvement make it a challenge, especially in low resource countries. Grossly, infectious uveitis is more common in LMICs, and autoimmune disorders-related uveitis is seen in high-income countries [1, 2].

For this perspective review chapter, a literature search was conducted on PubMed using the terms *uveitis* and *low- and middle-income countries*. The search yielded 21 results. After excluding 15 irrelevant articles, 6 were selected and reviewed for relevance and suitability. These included: a case report of infectious uveitis caused by tuberculosis [3]; two articles focusing on pediatric uveitis [4, 5]; a review discussing immune-mediated uveitis in the context of lifestyle factors [6]; one article addressing the use of systemic immunosuppressive therapies in developing countries [7]; and one study examining the pattern of uveitis in the Eastern Province of Saudi Arabia [8].

2. Global prevalence and incidence

It is estimated that more than 2 million people worldwide suffer from uveitis, and the number is increasing [9]. Geographical variations are seen in the prevalence and incidence of uveitis across the globe. Although the majority of the research and epidemiological studies are conducted in high-income countries, literature shows that it affects 38–200 individuals per 100,000, and incidence is reported as 17–52 individuals per 100,000 people [10]. About 25% of blindness in India and other developing countries is attributed to uveitis and its complications, such as secondary cataract, glaucoma, cystoid macular edema, or retinal photoreceptor or optic nerve damage [11]. Anterior uveitis is common in certain areas and posterior uveitis is common in other parts such as Africa. Whereas Japan and India have more cases of panuveitis. According to a West African study, Ebola-associated uveitis contributed to up to 2% of uveitis [12]. Data is limited regarding other types of uveitis due to limited epidemiological research in LMICs [13].

Data from high-income countries suggest that uveitis associated with autoimmune diseases and non-infectious uveitis is prevalent in these countries. Infectious uveitis is more common in LMICs. For example, Tuberculosis and Toxoplasmosis. This increased prevalence is largely attributed to limited healthcare resources and greater exposure to infectious agents. Healthcare expenditure in LMICs varies considerably, influenced by economic development, government priorities, and external funding sources. There are other reasons as well, which include environmental factors. For example, industrialization has improved human health through advancements in medical care and sanitation, leading to a decline in infectious diseases and infectious uveitis. However, it has also brought significant lifestyle changes, which have been increasingly linked to the development of various autoimmune diseases over the past decade. Presently, the lifestyle, hygiene standards, and environmental conditions differ markedly between developed and developing nations. The "lifestyle hypothesis" has been proposed to explain the variation in uveitis types between these regions. In developed countries, superior sanitation has lowered the incidence of infectious uveitis, while lifestyle changes may have contributed to a rise in immune-mediated forms. This disparity is likely to explain the differing proportions of immune-mediated uveitis observed between developed and developing countries.

3. Challenges of LMIC in managing uveitis

The barriers to eye care access comprise a long list, including economic, logistical, and educational factors.

3.1 Economic challenges

According to the World Bank reports, health expenditure per capita in LMICs is far short of that in high-income countries where it is more than $4000. Out of the national health budgets, a rudimentary amount is allocated to eye care. Most of the expenditures for eye care come from non-governmental organizations (NGOs) and international donors. Despite this external support, eye care spending falls short of the actual needs. This makes it very difficult to manage complicated conditions like uveitis.

3.2 Human resource challenges

Management of uveitis becomes a challenge when there are an average of 3.7 ophthalmologists per million in LMICs as compared to high-income countries where there is an average of 76.2 ophthalmologists per million individuals. The number is further lower for subspecialty consultants.

3.3 Diagnostic challenges

LMICs are facing diagnostic challenges due to a lack of infrastructure and limited diagnostic facilities, which is further complicated by the complex nature of the disease, which in some cases requires a series of diagnostic tests not easily available in LMICs. The challenge becomes manyfold with poor healthcare infrastructure, similarity of symptoms across different uveitis etiologies, and the need for expertise. There is also a high prevalence of infectious uveitis in LMICs, which requires specific diagnostic investigations and treatment protocols. The basic investigations, such as chest and sinus X-rays, chest computed tomography for sarcoidosis, magnetic resonance imaging, or positron emission tomography-computed tomography for vasculitis, are not available in peripheral areas. Unfortunately, there are no standard screening tests for uveitis. Advanced diagnostic tools, such as optical coherence tomography and fundus photography, are also available in tertiary care centers and are not accessible in remote areas, limiting the ability to accurately diagnose and monitor disease. While advanced diagnostic technologies exist, they are often too expensive for the poor population.

3.4 High prevalence of infectious diseases

Infectious diseases like tuberculosis and dengue require specific treatment protocols and diagnostic tests, such as polymerase chain reaction (PCR) on ocular fluids, which may not be readily available. The treatment has to be done on trial and error.

3.5 Systemic diseases as cause of uveitis

Approximately 25% of uveitis patients have associated systemic conditions [14]. One of the commonest infectious diseases associated with uveitis is Tuberculosis. Uveitis may be present with or without active TB. In some cases, a detailed systemic evaluation with collaboration with an internist is necessitated, especially in cases that fail to respond to empirical therapy and remain undiagnosed during acute episodes. A multidisciplinary approach is the key in such cases, with effective collaboration among different specialties. However, in LMICs, this is not easy. These countries are also affected by dangerous pathogens and outbreaks due to crowded conditions and limited medical facilities.

3.6 Lack of technological support in LMIC

Use of AI and teleophthalmology has helped in bridging the gap between remote areas and access to medical facilities. However, these technologies are far from being available in LMICs. While high-income countries are making use of technical support from smartphone-based visual acuity tests and portable imaging devices to be used by non-specialist healthcare providers in delivering effective eye care, such facilities are scarce in resource-constrained countries. Using technical staff and these sophisticated technical tools can offer some help in diagnosing and treating uveitis in remote areas of LMICs.

3.7 Barriers to eye care access

Physical distance from the eye care services, inadequate transportation, and limited insurance coverage add fuel to the already exhausted healthcare systems. The high cost of eye care services, coupled with limited insurance coverage, discourages many patients from seeking medical attention.

3.8 Educational barriers

Low literacy rate adds to the problems when patients, instead of seeking medical advice, go to the quacks for remedy. There is a lack of adequate training for local healthcare providers. Sometimes life threats to the healthcare workers multiply the problems. This results in delayed diagnosis and mismanagement. Traditional medicines and self-treatment complicate a usual case of uveitis, which contributes to the complexity of challenge.

3.9 Scarcity of local data for machine learning applications

Nowadays, machine learning can help in the early diagnosis of uveitis and other eye diseases with the use of large local datasets. In many LMICs, there is a lack of local data, which hinders the use of machine learning in these populations. Without local data, AI models do not prove to be as useful because of genetic, environmental, and epidemiological variations.

3.10 Treatment challenges

3.10.1 Limited access to medications

In uveitis, corticosteroids and immunosuppressive agents are the mainstay of the treatment in controlling inflammation and preventing complications. However, there are barriers to the high cost of medications, limited availability, and poor healthcare infrastructure. The disease is longstanding and requires long-term therapy, which leads to inconsistent treatment adherence and suboptimal disease control. This is complicated by the supply chain issues and other regulatory barriers, making access to the necessary medicines a nightmare. This often results in complications of uveitis, such as cataract and glaucoma or permanent vision loss. Poor policies further complicate drug affordability. Strengthening healthcare systems and expanding access to essential medications through government and non-government support and international collaborations can help address these issues.

3.10.2 Poor patient compliance

Patient compliance plays a major role in the management of diseases. In LMICs, patients' compliance and adherence are very poor owing to multiple factors including illiteracy, lack of disease awareness, and financial constraints. According to one study, non-compliance with treatment was observed in 22.4% of patients. The most frequently reported reasons included insufficient counseling by the treating physician, accounting for 26.7% of cases, and a demanding work or school schedule, reported by 22.2% of patients [15]. The follow-ups are inconsistent, leading to missed appointments and disease relapses and complications. Due to a lack of trust on the treating physicians, the medicines are discontinued owing to the side effects of corticosteroids and immunosuppressive drugs. On the ophthalmologists' part, counseling becomes difficult due to the heavy patient load in outpatient departments. The patients seek advice of quacks for traditional and alternative medicines, which is further strengthened by cultural beliefs. This requires patient education programs, strong healthcare initiatives, and community services to improve treatment adherence and disease outcomes.

3.10.3 Lack of national or regional uveitis management guidelines

For properly managing a disease based on the local situations, it is important to have standardized national and regional guidelines, which are not available in LMICs, creating a significant challenge in managing uveitis. There is a lack of consistent and evidence-based care, which results in variations in diagnosis, treatment, and patient outcomes. The following are some of the challenges faced due to the absence of local treatment protocols and guidelines:

- Due to a lack of proper protocols, every ophthalmologist struggles to find the best diagnostic and treatment approach, which can be based on trial and error, resulting in delayed diagnosis and complications. As the disease is variable in clinical presentations, some cases remain undiagnosed or misdiagnosed for a long time.

- LMICs have more prevalence of infectious uveitis. Without proper diagnosis, starting empirical treatments, such as corticosteroids, can be dangerous.

- Due to a lack of structured treatment protocols, treatment is not standardized, where some patients are overtreated and others are undertreated.

- Many ophthalmologists remain unaware of the newer biologic and immunomodulatory agents and stick to the steroids even in cases of no response.

- As there are no standardized guidelines, patients are not followed up at regular intervals, increasing the chances of glaucoma, cataracts, or vision loss.
- There is a disparity in treatment between the rural and urban areas and between the public and private setups.
- Healthcare providers in posh areas may follow the best international practices, but smaller hospitals and clinics lack resources. This may result in outdated management strategies.
- There is a knowledge and practice gap due to a lack of local guidelines affecting the outcomes of uveitis. This may result in unnecessary referrals, delayed diagnosis, and mismanagement.
- Resistance to anti-tubercular medicines had developed due to inadequate treatments [16].
- As there is no agreed-upon treatment, multicenter and national research is not possible.
- Lack of data further affects the development of evidence-based policies and resource allocation for uveitis care.

3.11 Challenges in making and implementing health reforms

Most of the LMICs lack management guidelines for uveitis, as discussed in the previous section. However, implementing already existing models and strategies is also not possible in the majority of areas. The following are the barriers in implementing health reforms:

3.11.1 Political and economic barriers

Unfortunately, many LMICs are politically unstable and face economic instability, resulting in limited funding and inadequate healthcare budgets, making it difficult to launch sustainable programs for uveitis management. This is further complicated by bureaucratic inefficiencies and inconsistent policies.

3.11.2 Human resource shortages

Management of uveitis requires a team of ophthalmologists, rheumatologists, internists, and other medical specialists. Shortage of trained specialist teams poses a critical challenge in uveitis management. In LMICs, the number of ophthalmologists per capita is very low, and subspecialty training in uveitis is often unavailable. This results in delayed diagnosis or misdiagnosis, delayed management, and often limited access to specialized treatments.

3.11.3 Educational gaps

Educational gaps at both the patient and doctor levels affect the implementation of policies. This requires state-level efforts to strengthen continuing professional development programs and patient education programs.

DOI: http://dx.doi.org/10.5772/intechopen.1010678

3.12 Challenges at primary eye care

Primary healthcare system in LMICs is in its infancy. Patients are bound to seek tertiary care services which are long distances from primary care. Strong primary healthcare services can help with early diagnosis and treatment, regular and accessible follow-up, and better management.

3.12.1 Weak integration of primary eye care services

Even in regions where primary healthcare services are better, they do not have adequate eye care services. General practitioners are not trained enough to diagnose uveitis at an early stage or to refer patients to specialists on time.

3.12.2 Barriers related to social factors

There are social factors which influence the management of uveitis at primary healthcare centers. Women are financially dependent with extra household responsibilities, and they have restrictions on mobility. Similarly, elderly patients are more vulnerable to eye diseases, but they face difficulties in seeking medical care. In some areas, minority populations are also underprivileged. This results in patients being presented at advanced stages of the disease, when treatment is less effective, and complications are more severe.

3.12.3 Overburdened specialized healthcare facilities

Being unsatisfied with the primary healthcare, people seek tertiary care as a last resort when complications have already occurred. This results in overburdened specialized hospitals where they face longer wait times and limited resources for advanced treatment.

4. Future directions

The challenges are huge, and resources are scarce. To address these challenges, a multi-pronged approach is necessary. The following are some general solutions to these issues:

4.1 Strengthening healthcare policies and systems

- Prioritize eye healthcare in policy making and allocate adequate funds.
- Develop standardized national and regional uveitis management guidelines.
- Expand insurance coverage and provide subsidies.

4.2 Enhancing diagnosis and treatment accessibility

- Invest in diagnostic tools.
- Promote teleophthalmology and AI-based screening.

- Promote the use of mHealth solutions for remote patient education, follow-ups, and medication adherence.

4.3 Increasing public awareness and community engagement

- Conduct educational campaigns at all levels to encourage early medical consultations and discourage self-medication.

- Train and help teachers and community workers in performing basic vision screenings, especially for children.

- Involve local stakeholders in building trust and improving healthcare.

4.4 Workforce development and capacity building

- Start training programs for general practitioners and community health workers to improve early uveitis detection.

- Offer workshops and digital learning platforms for healthcare providers.

- Encourage collaboration between researchers, healthcare providers, and policymakers to develop and distribute cost-effective diagnostic tools.

While these strategies show promise, challenges such as resource limitations and cultural barriers remain significant. Addressing these issues requires a multifaceted approach that combines technological innovation with community-based solutions. The following table summarizes a general framework on eye care integration for managing uveitis (**Table 1**).

	Challenges	Possible solution
1	Economic challenges	Targeted investment, global partnerships, and sustainable financing can help overcome economic barriers
2	Human resource challenges	Scaling up training, retention strategies, and equitable distribution can effectively address human resource shortages
3	Diagnostic challenges	Improving access to affordable, point-of-care technologies and strengthening laboratory networks can help overcome diagnostic challenges.
4	High Prevalence of Infectious Diseases	Enhancing preventive measures, vaccination programs, and public health education can significantly reduce the high prevalence of infectious diseases.
5	Systemic diseases as cause of uveitis	Integrating multidisciplinary care and early screening for systemic diseases can improve the diagnosis and management of uveitis
6	Lack of technological support in LMIC	Investing in scalable digital health solutions and infrastructure can bridge the technological gap
7	Barriers to Eye Care Access	Expanding community outreach, subsidized services, and mobile eye care units can effectively reduce barriers to eye care access.

	Challenges	Possible solution
8	Educational barriers	Implementing community-based health education and inclusive training programs
9	Scarcity of local data for machine learning applications.	Promoting local data collection initiatives and collaborative data-sharing platforms can mitigate the scarcity of local data for machine learning applications
10	Treatment Challenges	Improving access to medications, enhancing patient education for better compliance, and developing comprehensive national or regional uveitis management guidelines can address treatment challenges.
11	Challenges in Making and Implementing Health Reforms	Overcoming political and economic barriers, investing in workforce development, and addressing educational gaps through targeted policies can facilitate effective health reforms.
12	Challenges At Primary Eye Care	Strengthening the integration of primary eye care services, addressing social determinants of health, and improving the referral system can alleviate challenges at primary eye care levels.

Table 1.
Summary of the challenges in managing uveitis and possible solutions.

5. Clinical vignette

A 30-year-old lady presented to a tertiary care center with decreased vision in her right eye for 3 months. She was a village resident and had been under the treatment of quacks. She was the sole breadwinner for her family, working as a house cleaner in multiple homes to support her three children and care for her husband, who struggled with addiction. For the last 1one year, she noticed some blurry vision in her right eye but dismissed it as eye strain from daily chores and tiredness. When she started feeling pain in the eye, she resorted to the local healer who was a quack and prescribed her topical steroids. When her vision continued to worsen, her family turned to a spiritual healer who claimed her condition was due to an "evil eye" and

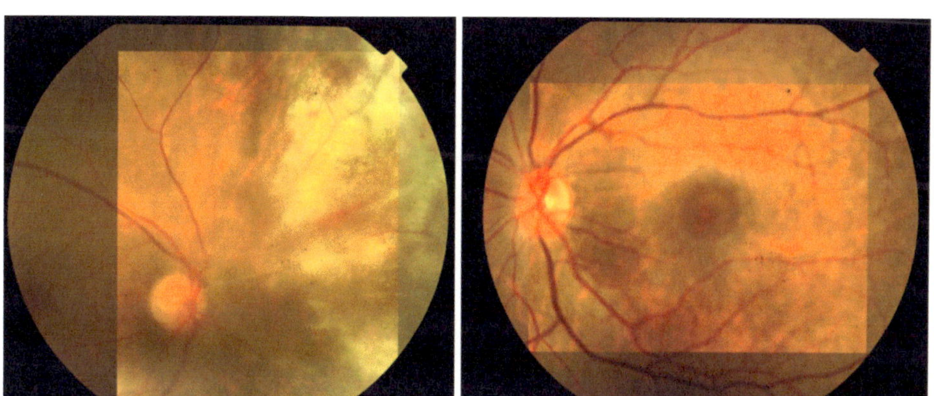

Figure 1.
Tuberculous uveitis in a 30-years old lady. Right eye shows vasculitis and posterior uveitis mostly involving nasal side of retina. Left eye is normal.

performed rituals to expel it. She was advised to stop medications and rely solely on spiritual remedies. The condition deteriorated. When a team of ophthalmologists visited the village for an eye camp, she was diagnosed with posterior uveitis. Her intraocular pressures were raised due to the continuous use of steroid eye drops. She was referred to a tertiary eye center, where she underwent treatment after investigations. Her Mantoux test was positive, and she was started on anti-tubercular therapy. The fundus picture of her right eye is shown in **Figure 1**. Her topical steroids were stopped and anti-glaucoma therapy started. Her story became a turning point for her community, highlighting the importance of early medical intervention and raising awareness about the dangers of relying on unqualified practitioners.

6. Conclusion

Uveitis is a significant global health concern. Its burden varies from LMICs to high-income countries. There are differences in healthcare infrastructure, economic resources, and disease epidemiology. LMICs face great challenges, including limited access to specialized care, lack of diagnostic facilities, and financial constraints, which hinder effective management of uveitis. There are barriers that should be overcome. It requires a multifaceted approach, starting from making healthcare reforms, strengthening primary eye care, decreasing illiteracy, improving health awareness, incorporating technology, and involving international community. Only then can uveitis-related blindness and disability be properly addressed.

Conflict of interest

The authors declare no conflict of interest.

Author details

Tayyaba Gul Malik[1*] and Noor Ul Ain[2]

1 Lahore General Hospital, Post Graduate Medical Institute, Ameer ud din Medical College, Lahore, Pakistan

2 Mughal Eye Hospital, Lahore, Pakistan

*Address all correspondence to: tayyabam@yahoo.com

References

[1] Prado KF, Couto LC, Moreira JE, Bontempo AS, Santos JL. Uveitis: Ocular manifestations of rheumatic diseases and multidisciplinary approaches. Brazilian Journal of Implantology and Health Science. 2024;**6**(5):956-968. DOI: 10.36557/2674-8169.2024v6n5p956-968

[2] Modrzejewska M, Zdanowska O, Świstara D. Current diagnostic options in uveitis–A review of the literature. Pomeranian Journal of Life Sciences. 2024;**70**(2). DOI: 10.21164/pomjlifesci.1017

[3] Nandu N, Bavanasi A, Wajahat R. Ocular tuberculosis without a lung primary. Cureus. 2020;**12**(5):e7920. DOI: 10.7759/cureus.7920

[4] Gentile P, Ragusa E, Bolletta E, De Simone L, Gozzi F, Cappella M, et al. Epidemiology of pediatric uveitis. Ocular Immunology and Inflammation. 2023;**31**(10):2050-2059. DOI: 10.1080/09273948.2023.2271988

[5] Abd El Latif E, Mousa R, Tawfeeq Mahdi M, Mahmoud Amin A, Mohammed Ahmed Ali M, Abdelhamid NE, et al. Etiology of pediatric uveitis in a tertiary pediatric eye hospital in Egypt. Ocular Immunology and Inflammation. 2023;**31**(10):1978-1983. DOI: 10.1080/09273948.2022.2117201

[6] Guo X, Chen Z, Xing Y. Immune-mediated uveitis and lifestyle factors: A review. Ophthalmic Research. 2021;**64**(5):687-695. DOI: 10.1159/000518496

[7] Agrawal H, Doan H, Pham B, Khosla A, Babu M, McCluskey P, et al. Systemic immunosuppressive therapies for uveitis in developing countries. Indian Journal of Ophthalmology. 2020;**68**:1852-1862

[8] Alarfaj G, Alahmadi G, Alabdullah H, Al-Khars W, Al-Hammad F. Pattern of uveitis at a tertiary eye hospital in eastern province of Saudi Arabia and comparison with local literature. Ocular Immunology and Inflammation. 2023;**31**(9):1837-1841. DOI: 10.1080/09273948.2022.2128822

[9] Foster CS, Kothari S, Anesi SD, Vitale AT, Chu D, Metzinger JL, et al. The ocular immunology and uveitis foundation preferred practice patterns of uveitis management. Survey of Ophthalmology. 2016;**61**(1):1-17

[10] García-Aparicio Á, García de Yébenes MJ, Otón T, Muñoz-Fernández S. Prevalence and incidence of uveitis: A systematic review and meta-analysis. Ophthalmic Epidemiology. 2021;**28**(6):461-468. DOI: 10.1080/09286586.2021.1882506

[11] Rao NA. Uveitis in developing countries. Indian Journal of Ophthalmology. 2013;**61**(6):253-254. DOI: 10.4103/0301-4738.114090

[12] Balendra S, Harrison-Williams L, Mustapha J, Koroma Z, Kamara A, Saradugu B, et al. Clinical characteristics and aetiology of uveitis in a viral haemorrhagic fever zone. Eye (London, England). 2024;**38**(11):2110-2116. DOI: 10.1038/s41433-024-03009-0

[13] Miserocchi E, Fogliato G, Modorati G, Bandello F. Review on the worldwide epidemiology of uveitis. European Journal of Ophthalmol. 2013;**23**(5):705-717. DOI: 10.5301/ejo.5000278

[14] Barisani-Asenbauer T, Maca SM, Mejdoubi L, Emminger W, Machold K, Auer H. Uveitis-a rare disease often associated with systemic diseases and infections-a systematic review of 2619 patients. Orphanet Journal of Rare Diseases. 2012;7:1-7. DOI: 10.1186/1750-1172-7-57

[15] Patil A, Gupta S, Venkatesh P, Banerjee M, Kumar V, Chawla R, et al. First contact investigations and compliance to treatment in patients with uveitis. International Journal of Ophthalmology. 2023;**16**(11):1820-1826. DOI: 10.18240/ijo.2023.11.13

[16] Agrawal R, Gunasekeran DV, Grant R, Agarwal A, Kon OM, Nguyen QD, et al. Collaborative ocular tuberculosis study (COTS)–1 study group. Clinical features and outcomes of patients with tubercular uveitis treated with antitubercular therapy in the collaborative ocular tuberculosis study (COTS)-1. JAMA Ophthalmology. 2017;**135**(12):1318-1327. DOI: 10.1001/jamaophthalmol.2017.4485. Erratum in: JAMA Ophthalmol.2019;137(2):233. doi:10.1001/jamaophthalmol.2017.6239